ENDORSEMENTS

I've had the pleasure of knowing and working with Dr. Charlie Cole since 2012. His imagination, vision, and confidence is an inspiration to all. By creating a patient-centered, caring environment, he was able to grow his practice from zero revenue to a seven-figure business. His book offers invaluable advice for any practice owner looking to grow business and make a positive impact.

**WADE L. REED, CEO AT EXCEPTIONAL EXPERIENCES, INC,
A CUSTOMER/EMPLOYEE EXPERIENCE FIRM**

The Same Day Dentistry Revolution is a must-read for all dentists. With his transparent style, Dr. Cole shows how to transform your practice with his outside-the-box thinking. This step-by-step guide with Charlie's "Triple Win Strategies" will skyrocket your production, profitability, and put the fun back into dentistry.

THOMAS LAMBERT DDS, LECTURER, (KOL) KEY OPINION LEADER

T0098562

In his new book, Charlie Cole shows us that when you intentionally do good work, people will find and reward you. The world needs more professionals like him, who live out their values and put their hearts into everything they do.

BERNADETTE JIWA
BEST-SELLING BUSINESS AUTHOR
BRAND STORY & MARKETING STRATEGIST

It's crazy to think that Dr. Cole has found the secret to patient loyalty by offering a same day approach to dentistry. As a business consultant, we advocate for quality service and transparency of fees. He seems to have mastered both!

PAULA BRADISON, FOUNDER
SENIOR CONSULTANT OPERATIONS AND STRATEGY,
BRADISON MANAGEMENT GROUP

The Same Day Dentistry Revolution

THE
SAME DAY
DENTISTRY
REVOLUTION

The Path to a More Profitable,
Efficient and Enjoyable Experience
for You, Your Staff and Your Patients

CHARLIE COLE, DDS

NEW YORK

NASHVILLE • MELBOURNE • VANCOUVER

The Same Day Dentistry Revolution

The Path to a More Profitable, Efficient and Enjoyable Experience for You, Your Staff and Your Patients

Published in New York, New York, by Morgan James Publishing. Morgan James is a trademark of Morgan James, LLC. www.MorganJamesPublishing.com

The Morgan James Speakers Group can bring authors to your live event. For more information or to book an event visit The Morgan James Speakers Group at www.TheMorganJamesSpeakersGroup.com.

ISBN 9781683503521 paperback
ISBN 9781683503545 eBook
Library of Congress Control Number: 2016918827

Cover Design by:
Rachel Lopez
www.r2cdesign.com

Interior Design by:
Chris Treccani
www.3dogdesign.net

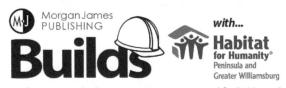

In an effort to support local communities, raise awareness and funds, Morgan James Publishing donates a percentage of all book sales for the life of each book to Habitat for Humanity Peninsula and Greater Williamsburg.

Get involved today! Visit
www.MorganJamesBuilds.com

CONTENTS

CHAPTER ONE

Dentistry on the Same Day? What's *That* All About?

I want to talk about two things: disruption and dentistry.

When you talk about disruption, dentistry probably isn't the next word that comes to mind. But I want to get us started off on the same level, and on that level, we're thinking a little differently.

We're thinking about how to make change, and for the better. We're thinking about problems that need solutions.

1

We're thinking about throwing out the playbook and starting from scratch.

More important—*most* important—here on this wavelength, we're thinking about being true to ourselves. For me, a dentist with decades of experience in traditional dental practices, being true to myself meant bringing a little of that disruption into dentistry. It meant starting the Same Day Dentistry revolution.

You might have been practicing the traditional model of dentistry for years too, owning your own practice and trying to make ends meet by keeping a rotating roster of ever-complicated procedures. Or, you might be a junior dentist, just starting out in your field and trying to scrape together a living working for different corporate dental centers throughout the week, worrying about paying off your school debt and supporting a young family. Or you might be a patient, frustrated by having to come back for procedure after procedure until you've crossed everything off your expensive treatment plan.

Make no mistake: I have no quarrel with the traditional way of doing things. And the way that I run my practice isn't for everyone, either. There's a time and a place for each type of treatment. But I wrote this book because the time might be right for a little revolution in your life too.

What We Do

It's as simple as it sounds: the Same Day Dentistry revolution is about performing dental procedures on the same day. Efficiently solving problems, being a dependable and trusted presence in patients' lives, helping them to get out of pain and move on with their day: that's what has driven me as a dentist for more than thirty-five years, and that's what we aim to do in a Same Day Dentistry practice.

Let's walk through it with a patient. We'll call him John. John has wandered in to my practice largely because he's seen our sign out front (we're located in a central strip mall, not a place you'd expect to find a dental practice, but we'll get to that later) and he's heard of us through positive word of mouth or social media. He's busy, he's scared, and he's in a *lot* of pain. The first thing I do is sit down with him for a one-on-one conversation; I gather his patient history, but more important, I listen for the type of experiences that he's had walking into dental practices before.

I can tell that John is feeling a little guilty and embarrassed. He's never particularly liked going to the dentist, he admits, and so that makes it hard for him to prioritize his dental care. I can't hold that against him; it's an intimidating prospect, letting a stranger poke around in your mouth with all those sharp implements! He's typically ignored problems in his mouth before, hoping they would go away.

"I have bad teeth," he explains, like it's something that is his fault, and then goes on to tell me about the last time he visited a dentist, two years ago.

He had a nagging toothache, one that he worried was the result of a cavity or an infection. He found a dentist on his insurance plan and went in for a consultation, hoping to get the problem addressed. He received a cursory exam and X-rays for a hefty out-of-pocket fee, and a treatment plan with an intimidating (and costly) list of issues to address.

"I have bad teeth," he says again.

Because he hadn't had the money that day for the entire treatment plan, he'd felt it wasn't worth starting down that road. He'd had a toothache *that day*, but he had walked out of that office with nothing but a hole in his bank account from the examination fees.

My first aim was to make sure that this didn't happen to John again. I knew that in the intervening years, some problems may have gotten worse—and some new decay had probably popped up. But I wanted to make sure that, no matter what, John would walk away with some sort of a solution *today*.

"So what brings you in today, John?"

"Well, I have a toothache."

The idea behind Same Day Dentistry is that we've set up our practice in such a way that we can offer same-day solutions. It's not that we turn away patients like John, who may have multiple needs to address over time. Instead, it's that we've made sure that patients like John can come in and get their most urgent needs addressed right then and there, with no added pressure to follow an overwhelming treatment plan (and no added pressure on us to have to sell him on that plan to meet our expenses).

Skeptics will decry that mission as unreasonable, but I beg to differ. By adhering to a policy of simplicity and transparency—clearly listing our services and their costs from the get-go on our website, in the waiting room, on all of our materials—we approach each patient with a clarity of purpose and a shared expectation of what the goals of treatment are for that visit. We're not trying to be all things to all people. It *would* be unreasonable to say that we could perform some complicated, multiday procedures in one day. Because one of the keys to the Same Day Dentistry revolution is that transparency and truth in process, we make it very clear what we can offer (exams, fillings, cleanings, sealants, crowns, implants, root canals, and removals, to name a few of our services) and what we can't.

So after listening to John's story, my first order of business is to get him in my chair to identify his problem and deliver a solution. I'm not thinking about what's going to happen down the road, worrying about whether or not John will return for the other procedures that he might need. Because I'm focused on providing excellent same-day solutions for John's most urgent issues, I know that the follow-up visits will take care of themselves. He came to us based on the strength of our good reputation, after all—on the trust that we've built over years in our community. And I'm banking that good reputation will only continue into the future after we've solved some problems for John in the present.

How We Do It

For me, it all comes back to that belief in the Same Day Dentistry mission. My entire office is attuned to it; everyone from my office manager to my dental assistants understands what we're trying to achieve, and we're all committed to that one goal: providing superior service and making people feel better that same day.

To believe in this mission *in theory* is one thing, but to *put it into practice* is another. I'm incredibly fortunate to have a team that is willing to walk the walk. It's not a philosophy that would fly in most offices; if you call your dental office at 4:00 p.m. and they close at 4:30 p.m., you probably will expect to be told by the receptionist that you can't be seen until the next day. In our office, the approach is different. "How about tomorrow?" becomes "How soon can you get here?"

Same Day Dentistry might remind you of an urgent care clinic in that respect, and I'm OK with that comparison. If you've ever had something go wrong in your mouth when the clock is ticking toward the end of a workday, you know that feeling of dread that comes with the idea that you might not be able to find relief until the following business day—and that's in the best-case scenario. To me, there's not much that seems more urgent than that. My staff feels the same way.

And, ultimately, it's that level of customer service that makes me comfortable shrugging off the outdated model of having patients essentially on retainer. Everyone who comes in to our office is a Same Day Dentistry patient the first time he or she comes in. That doesn't mean that it's the only time we'll see that patient—far from it, in fact. We've grown our repeat business substantially over two years, scheduling patients for return visits based on the same premise on which we treated them the first time they walked through our door. No matter what we're scheduling them for in the future, they'll always know that the return visit will be of the same quality, the same timeliness, the Same Day Dentistry way.

Whereas the traditional model of dentistry might pressure you to close cases bringing in $4,000 to $6,000 of dentistry at a time, at the end of the day, the numbers that actually get pulled in aren't that impressive. If you have the rates of a typical dental practice, you're probably closing about 20 percent of those cases. But with the Same Day Dentistry model, you're establishing trust faster, you're solving problems more immediately, and you're closing cases at a much higher rate.

Why We Do It

First and foremost, the Same Day Dentistry revolution is designed to benefit the people who make our jobs worthwhile: the patients. Being able to see someone come into my office, sit down, and leave later that day free from the pain of an infected tooth or with the benefits of a new smile thanks to implants? That's priceless to me. Above all else, I believe that a good dentist must be motivated by patient care. Quality dental care affects quality of life.

But there's another group of people I'm hoping to help by spreading the word about Same Day Dentistry: my fellow dental professionals. This became particularly evident to me as I was in an interview to hire a junior dentist to join my practice, which has grown tremendously over the past three years (so much so, in fact, that I need to scale up my staff to keep our Same Day Dentistry promise).

I went into the interview with a young associate who, at four years out of dental school, was being stretched a little thin. He had a young family, and was cobbling together an existence working on an hourly rate at a few different big, corporate dental centers. Six days a week, he found himself splitting time between three offices, trying—and failing—to make a dent in paying off his school debt.

I could see right away that this was a man who loved the profession. I could see something of myself in him: the psychological struggle he was enduring as he watched traditional dental practices rife with inefficiencies fall short of the ideals that he had once had when he'd started off on this journey. And I could see that, like many of us when we're just starting out in life, he didn't necessarily know there was a world apart from the one into which he had been indoctrinated. He probably assumed that all jobs would be like those first jobs, that all offices would be run the same way.

After touring our office, we sat down together to talk over what he'd seen. He lauded our office's efficiency, our organization, our approach, and so on.

"There's no way I could do the amount of dentistry you're able to do in a day," he said. "It's mind-blowing."

I was so proud to hear him say that, to know that his mind had been opened to the possibility that there was another approach, a different way to conduct dentistry. But I knew I had to disabuse him of the notion that it wasn't something that could be replicated with the right approach. I felt it was my duty to tell him that he didn't have to be locked into the world of corporate dentistry, into the management principles that have served my generation for years but which are totally out of sync with the way that we live our lives now. That he, too, could earn the kind of living that he had thought possible when he'd enrolled in dental school— not just in the financial sense, but in the sense of holding down a rewarding job that also allowed him some time to breathe and enjoy his young family. That we were no different and that I was in his place not too long ago.

Maybe the Same Day Dentistry approach will be right for our junior dentist. Maybe not. Maybe it'll be right for your practice, or maybe it won't. I have no qualms with the traditional model. I just knew it wasn't right *for me*. And if I can give a little bit of that insight to you—as a provider, as a patient, as a *person*—then I'll feel like I have done my job. I'll feel like I've opened your mind to the possibility of thinking differently. As with my patients, I know that something brought you here today. Something brought you to this book.

I'm so glad you're here, and I'm hoping that you're going to like what you read.

CHAPTER TWO

From Someday to Same Day
How the Whole Thing Came About

I f I were to trace back to the beginning of the Same Day Dentistry Revolution, I'd have to say it's probably been more of an *evolution* than anything else—something that I gradually came to over time. Having practiced conventional dentistry for quite some time, I'd seen some places here and there along the way that could benefit from efficiencies or changes—things I'd keep in the back of my mind for that magical "someday," whenever that happened to come along. But for the most part, I was just perpetuating the cycle that I'd been taught. That's how the status quo becomes status quo, after all.

Throughout my time in the industry, I purchased and sold three businesses, all told. Following the model that was held up as an example for me during my training, I would purchase a practice that has cash flow and a patient roster, then do what I could to dress it up a bit: a little marketing here, a little office renovation there. But I found myself slipping into the role of my predecessor: picking up his demeanor, his style of dentistry, his way of doing things. There seemed to be little room for that idea of staying true to myself that I talked about in the first chapter.

Predictably, things would hit a plateau from there, and I wouldn't be too satisfied. Thinking it was time to shake things up, I'd sell the practice and repeat the whole process again, ignoring that old adage about the definition of insanity: it's really just doing the same thing again and again, all the while, expecting a different result. And the financial side wasn't much different; not only was I not getting personal fulfillment from perpetuating this old model, but I also wasn't left with much to show for my work when all was said and done and the accounts and taxes were settled after each sale.

So the way things worked wasn't working for me anymore. But like many experienced business owners, I was between that proverbial rock and a hard place: too young to retire and too invested in my career path to totally start over. I knew that I wasn't ready to leave dentistry. There were still things—my patients, chief among them—that I very much still loved about dentistry. But where could I go from there?

In life, as in so many of the rich fables that hold life's lessons, a deus ex machina often bursts onto the scene. Ready to destroy everything in its path, a fire-breathing monster comes down upon the kingdom. But the wonderful thing about fire and destruction is that in its wake, it often leaves rich, fertile soil. It leaves room for growth. It leaves opportunity.

This was certainly the case, although I didn't exactly know it at the time, when I found myself getting fired around Christmastime in 2013. I had been working as an associate at another dentist's practice as my backup plan; I was in the midst of selling my third dental practice. In between hours at the office, I had been casting about for a better way forward in my career, talking with a consulting group about the possibility of opening up a nonprofit dental center much in the model of the Mayo Clinic. So after I got over the initial shock of being blindsided by the blow to my fallback plan, I found myself looking firmly forward.

As it happened, the pink slip in my stocking turned out to be a gift instead of a curse. After a good deal of discussion and trepidation, talking for hours at a time with my wife and a dental consulting firm that really took an interest in me as a person, as opposed to trying to plug me into a tried (and tired) formula, I had a new plan.

And boy, was it scary.

That plan was to be the beginning of the revolution.

The revolution would start with me building my own practice from the ground up. That meant no steady cash flow to coast in on, no existing patient roster to act as a security blanket. Rather than buying another dentist's practice, I was giving myself the opportunity to start fresh, and to build the practice around my ideals.

Just two short months after I had woken up wondering *"What's next?"* the first piece of the puzzle came into focus when I found a building that used to be a medical facility nestled inside an unassuming strip mall in Wasilla, Alaska. I spent from February to July of that year acquiring the space, cleaning it out, and tidying it up, getting it ready for the vision of what I thought my patients' needs would be, and for what *my* needs would be. First and foremost was the need to stay true to myself.

Nearly a decade ago, I started looking for my true north. Geographically, that ended up being Alaska; I had spent some time there in the 1980s, and after running dental practices in the Midwest and seeing my children through high school and college, I was drawn back to the state's rugged beauty. But more than just finding a home for myself, I was looking to salve a gnawing feeling I had inside.

We all waste so much time and energy trying to be something that we're not. Whether it's pressure from our families or society, or just a preconceived notion we have of what it means to be successful and worthy, there's a constant push and pull between ideals and reality, between the person we think we should be and the person we truly are. In the medical and dental professions, this often translates to high overheads, big bank accounts, fast cars, and high-flying planes.

That might be someone else's life, but it wasn't meant to be mine.

Still, standing in the empty office space one night before we opened, I couldn't help but feel more than a little afraid. There was no safety net, no status quo to fall back on. If I failed, the failure would be entirely on my shoulders; there would be no predecessor to blame and no security blanket in which to swaddle myself. Can you blame me?

But soon, that trepidation was eclipsed by the incredible sense of opportunity I felt. I took a moment to think about what being true to myself really meant. I thought about how I would structure my patient visits to align with those principles. Closing my eyes and standing on the quiet floor, I could see it.

Years prior, I had gotten a taste of what the Same Day Dentistry revolution might look like when I invested in a CAD/CAM crown machine that was able to make crowns in one day. I saw how efficient the system was, and how happy patients were when they could have an entire procedure performed in the same day rather than having to return for multiple follow-ups. For the patient, it eliminated the pain and inconvenience of post-op visits, and for me and my staff, it eliminated the concern that we'd have patients failing to come to those visits for budgetary or personal reasons. This allowed us, in turn, to reduce our fees, saving the patient even more money in the end.

I wanted to apply that kind of ease and efficiency to everything that I would do in this new practice, and I imagined what that might look like. A new patient would come in; after all, from the start, everyone would be a new patient. I knew I'd want to personally greet him and sit down with him face-to-face rather than having him waiting vulnerably in a dental chair from the get-go. And I would listen, *truly* listen, when he answered my first and only question: "What can we do for you *today?*"

It might be an aching tooth or a loose filling. Inevitably, other issues might arise, and that was OK. I'd let the patient know that we would deal with those when he was ready to, always keeping the focus on his chief concern: the thing that had brought him into my office *that day.* I'd take the time to develop a relationship with my patient rather than inundating him with a long, expensive treatment plan. Under no circumstances would I rush the relationship, because I knew that building a strong foundation was essential to bringing him back for repeat visits.

But more than that, being true to myself meant that I could sleep at night with a clear conscience and the bone-deep satisfaction of a job well done. Not because I was thinking of those repeat visits as a way to make my payroll—although I don't want to downplay the importance of having a viable business model—but rather, because the relationships I was building would ultimately let my patients receive better, more comprehensive dental care. Being true to myself meant making sure I was being true to my patients.

Whether or not you wind up implementing the Same Day Dentistry revolution, I would encourage you to take some time out of your day to think about what being true to yourself means, and also, what being true to your patients means. What do your patients really need? I've watched my patients' needs change over the past few decades; we're living in a culture that's moving at a faster pace. We're living in an economy that demands that most households have both parents working full-time jobs, meaning, the parent responsible for childcare is taking time away from *two* jobs if he or his children need dental attention. So, for me, it was even *more* important to develop a model of dentistry where we could save patients time, money, and hopefully even a little sanity!

At the end of my reflection upon the blank slate of what would become Same Day Dentistry, I opened my eyes. I wasn't sure of what the future would hold. But I knew that whatever it would look like, my aim would be true.

I can't say for certain, but I'm pretty sure I slept soundly that night.

From Flying Blind to Flying to Paradise

When we started from scratch, it was just me and an office manager. In under three years, we grew to two front-of-office folks, three dental assistants, and one dental hygienist—and I'm working on bringing a junior dentist on board, in addition to training more dental assistants. But when I say it was a small shop when we got going, I mean it, and we had a patient base to match.

I worked on generating all the good will I could. And thankfully, we'd had a captive audience all those months we were working with local contractors and designers who helped us bring the office together on time and under budget. I gave free dental care to everyone who helped me remodel the office: the plumbers, the electricians, the drywallers, the manager of the strip mall that would become our new home. I wanted to pay them back for all their help, but selfishly, I knew that the best way for news of our services to trickle out would be to start on a grassroots level. And it worked remarkably well. I can still recall working on the man who installed our telephones; to this day, he's been one of my most valuable advocates.

In those early days, we did spend a lot of time hoping that the phone would ring. I took a job working as a dentist at a prison in the area, relieving some of the financial pressure that I had created by stepping out on my own, and getting my name out in the community as a result. I'd like to say that my skill as a dentist has contributed to all of this positive word-of-mouth advertising, but if I stopped there, I'd be overlooking an important factor—one of the driving principles behind the business, in fact.

Simply put, I think that *transparency* plays a huge role in creating the positive buzz that has surrounded Same Day Dentistry for the past three years—putting ourselves out there (literally, in an easy-to-find commercial location), building relationships, giving people an approachable and honest practice to turn to.

We've got nothing to hide, and it shows. We post our list of services and prices right on our window and on our website. Our reception areas have no walls, no barriers. In contrast to most dental offices, where the waiting area occupies a tiny corner of the office before it turns into a maze of walls and rooms, we've built a practice that welcomes patients from the moment they walk in the door.

That's the way that felt most natural for me from the standpoint of creating a practice that was true to my values, but that kind of transparency is essential for any business in this day and age of social media and instantaneous feedback. If you fail to be authentic and transparent, that negative feedback can quickly go viral. But on the other side of the coin, the power of a good review can be multiplied many times over once social media comes into play. Authentic advertising is priceless.

That authenticity also saves me the pain of trying to wear another hat that doesn't quite fit. I'm no salesman; I never have been, and I never want to be. By building my practice around solving patient problems rather than padding my bank account, I've ensured a financially stable future without having to compromise my objectives. I've found that if you give patients what they came for, the services aren't a hard sell, and that when I'm less focused on selling, I can be more focused on what really matters to me: the patient.

Three years and a lot of learning later, I'm nowhere near done with my work. But I am done trying to be someone who I'm not. And, thankfully, I'm also done with worrying each day about whether or not I'll make my payroll. Never in my wildest dreams would I have thought it would be possible to make a viable business based on a nontraditional model. I'm so happy to say that I dream bigger now, cushioned by the large amount of cash flow we can count on daily as a result of our same-day services.

Never would I have thought that we would come so far from that night when I was standing in the empty office thinking about the risk I was about to take. In fact, it wasn't really until two and a half years into this journey, as I was sitting on a beach in Turks and Caicos and enjoying a prepaid, all-inclusive vacation with my wife and my entire staff, that I really started to breathe a little easier, to feel like I'd finally found my true north.

CHAPTER THREE

Why the Traditional Model of Selling Dentistry Is Broken

L et's take a field trip, shall we?

Pretend for a moment that you're sitting in a park on your lunch break, only a mile away from your office. You've released yourself from the grip of the sad desk lunch and you're enjoying some fresh air for once. All is right with the world. But suddenly, you hear a hiss coming from behind you in the parking lot. You turn to see that one of your front tires, which has been looking worn out for a little while now, finally just bit the dust.

It's not necessarily surprising; money's been tight and your car hasn't been your top priority while you've been trying to make ends meet, but it's still frustrating nonetheless, especially since you need to get back to work soon.

You've got a donut tire in the boot of your car, so you Google a local company to have someone come out to change the tire, thinking that once you've made it through the rest of the workday, you can drive the short distance from your office to your home and deal with the rest of the issue on your personal time.

Time passes—too much time, it turns out; you're already going to have to explain your long lunch break to the boss. But finally, a wrecker truck rounds the corner, and you couldn't be more relieved. You point to the obviously flat tire, and wait as patiently as you can while the mechanic ambles around the car, his expression becoming graver as he goes along.

It's not until he's got the car jacked up and your tire halfway off before he delivers his assessment.

"You've got a lot of problems here," he starts. "Your bearings are going out on that left rear tire, one of your lug nuts is stripped, and your brake pads look pretty burned-out right here."

You immediately feel sheepish, like you're being judged. *This guy's an expert in autos,* you think, *and here I am, showing him my junker in all its neglected glory.*

"Yeah," you admit, "I've been meaning to take care of that stuff. It has been vibrating a little bit. I'll definitely do that soon. But I really need to get back to work, so if you could just put the donut tire on, that would be great."

Just after you'd thought things couldn't get worse, he says: "Oh, and I see a leak in the rear transmission here. When's the last time you had this thing serviced?"

"Probably a year ago," you volunteer.

"Well, that's a problem. You're supposed to do that every four thousand miles. Get the oil checked, all that."

At this point, you can kiss good-bye a productive afternoon at work. You start to mentally tally up all the work the car needs and wonder where you're going to get the money. Then things continue to go downhill, and not because you're driving there.

"I really can't do anything for you right now," says the mechanic. "I could lose my license if I let you roll out of this parking lot and you get into an accident. I'm going to have to lift the car up on the back here and take it to the shop and do a full work-over."

That's bad enough. But this field trip isn't over. It turns out that since he isn't giving you much of a choice, you can't even have the donut tire put on, and just when you think the worst that's going to happen is that you'll have to be even later to work because you now have to call a friend to come help you out, he puts his hand out for his fee.

"It's your decision if you don't want the work done," he says, his hand outstretched, "but that'll still be $200 for all the diagnostic work I just put in here."

Nightmare, right?

Lucky for you, this is just a hypothetical situation! But the unfortunate truth is that this kind of experience is not too far from what patients have reported to me regularly when they talk about why they haven't been to the dentist in months, or even *years*, despite some pretty serious mouth pain.

The System Is Broken and So Is Their Trust

The way that traditional dentistry works right now is largely similar. A patient comes in for an initial visit. The dentist charges for a cursory examination and X-rays and then builds a treatment plan on top of that. If things are fairly straightforward—say, it's a new patient visit with no cavities or any trouble areas to report—the patient can go home with the satisfaction that he's entered a pipeline of care and can go about his business as usual, returning for two appointments per year, max.

But if things are more complicated—if there's a lot of work to be done, just as there was on that hypothetical car—the presentation of the treatment plan will likely do little more than just scare the patient away from the office for good, either for financial reasons, psychological reasons, or both. And, because dentists can easily bill insurance companies for this initial visit and they are concerned about recouping their expenses—particularly because the patient might not seem like he'll be returning, they charge the patient their visit fee anyway.

At the end of the day, they may feel a little guilty about not being able to do anything to help the patient, but since they are also human and feel the sting of rejection just as anyone would, they tell themselves, "You know, he just didn't appreciate quality dentistry. I don't want those patients anyway."

This makes me sad! It makes me sad because I sympathize with dentists who have pressure to make payroll and who have to go through the emotional pain of rejection. It makes me sad because I feel for patients who are in *physical* pain and can't get the help they need. And it makes me sad because those same patients will likely continue to neglect their dental health—something that, as ample medical evidence has shown, should be far from an optional expense!

As you may have gathered from this book's first chapters, I don't have a lot of patience for bad feelings at this point in my career. I decided I wanted to do something to change all that, and so I've done it in my new practice.

The patients aren't broken; the system is!

One thing I've experienced in my journey to the Same Day Dentistry way of doing things is that—and I'm making a generalization here—we dentists aren't really business masterminds. To help fill in the knowledge gap, we bring in consultants. But consultants have some of the same quandaries dentists have—and oftentimes, to keep their business going, they end up telling us what we want to hear. In my case and in the case of many others, what we want to hear is that we'll be secure, that we aren't risking everything, and that we're going to be able to handle our payroll and make a cushy salary on top of that.

But that security can be based on some false premises. For one, a dentist often measures his security on how full his calendar is. A schedule filled up months in advance gives a dentist a sense that he can project his cash flow and expenses months—even quarters—out. But the reality is that this schedule can change dynamically day to day. Patients get sick, their cars break down, they get laid off, they forget to come in.

By contrast, the Same Day Dentistry model can seem pretty scary. You may have some regular appointments on the books, but there's a lot of empty space on your calendar, and you might not be sure what the week, or even the day, may hold. It can take a relatively major shift in thinking to become comfortable with feeling confident that the number of walk-ins, emergencies, and other appointments will generate a tremendous amount of revenue (not to mention follow-ups, if the patient is impressed with your work!).

After three years, I've found that I'm averaging about $4,000 *a day* of walk-in treatment on top of our scheduled appointments.

But the problem goes further back than relying on consultants. When we train dentists in dental school, we're asking them to commit to diagnosing an incredible level of detail. This isn't the fault of dental schools; I don't know anyone who would want a dentist who was anything less than thorough. But what I mean to say is that *of course* dentists are predisposed to look at the entire picture. Then, because of how billing works and how much economic pressure there is for us to make payroll, we're translating that thorough diagnosis into a case plan that absolutely overwhelms patients.

Instead, I'm advocating for a different patient-relationship model. I'm advocating for getting to know your patient and making a plan born out of compassion, concern, and care. I'm not advocating ignoring larger problems or more complex issues, but I *am* advocating both a triage of finances and treatment to address the most pressing concern first in order to relieve a patient's pain. This, in turn, creates trust. And trust creates a meaningful foundation on which a relationship can be built.

Unlike the hypothetical mechanic who ultimately did more harm than help in the scenario at the start of the chapter, practitioners of the Same Day Dentistry revolution take a different tack. For the person who has the broken tooth, or the toothache, or whatever the problem is, I make a special effort to focus on the main concern first. And that means truly listening, not thinking ahead or trying to manipulate or upsell the patient. Because even though most dentists who do that are just perpetuating a system they've been trained in, and are genuinely trying to be helpful, what ends up happening is that patients walk away insulted, embarrassed, and still in pain.

Same Day Dentistry: A Better Way

So how do we approach this better way to dental care? It's not that our examination is any less thorough—we take the same X-rays and make the same list of everything we see in the exam—but it's less *pressure* for the patient. We have an orchestrated approach, one that always circles back to the main concern.

We'll get into the nitty-gritty of what to expect when you're a Same Day Dentistry patient in an upcoming chapter, but now I want to disabuse readers of any notion that we offer anything less than complete, thorough, and quality care. We share the results of the scans and exam with our patients, but only after we've thoroughly discussed their main concerns and gone through treatment options for those concerns. Anything that comes after that, we've asked their permission to discuss. And because we've earned their trust by clarifying our intentions to solve their most pressing problems, I generally find that I'm met with much less resistance than I would be otherwise.

If they're interested in hearing about the rest of their mouth, I take them through my findings. I explain in very plain terms how problems might worsen down the line, just as I walk them through the specifics of why we can afford to probably let some things wait, if that's what they need to do. I always go at their pace, and I remove any possibility of pressure or upselling by making it clear that unless they ask for anything further, we're only concentrating on the chief complaints that day. You can see the relief wash over them. Even when they're faced with a litany of cavities, they feel they've found someplace to take care of their dental health, and so an overwhelming list of issues to tackle in the future suddenly might not seem so daunting.

I also remove myself from the room before they have to come to any financial decisions, thereby distinguishing myself as a caregiver and distancing myself from any hint of salesmanship. The next time they see me, I'm going to be there to enact whatever course of treatment they've decided on. They know I won't be back to argue, and they know they won't be in for any other surprises.

It's not that patients don't *want* quality dental care. It's that there are logistical barriers: finance, time, even emotions. By focusing on building trust and asking patients for their permission to discuss further options for care, we're dismantling the emotional barriers. By not charging initial-exam fees and providing transparent, flat rates for services, we're easing the financial barriers. What's more, if you're selling someone something that he or she truly needs and wants, nothing is too expensive. Finally, by committing to solving patients' chief concerns in the same day, we're shattering those time barriers.

No Fees for the First Visit? Are You Nuts!?

One of the major areas in which I get pushback from other dental professionals on the Same Day Dentistry concept isn't time or treatment plans. It's money. Specifically, the money that my office "gives up" by declining to charge patients the typical fees for first exams and X-rays.

To those dentists who can't quite get on board with the idea, it seems as though I'm giving up an easy $200 to $600 of billing per patient, with that policy. When you're talking about the status quo of the system, especially where insurance

Step Out of Your Comfort Zone . . . and Into Success

I'm not sure if it's the way we're trained, or the way dentists and medical professionals are seen in society. I don't know if it's the lab coat or the honorific "Dr." But whatever the cause, there's an undeniable separation between dentist and patient. It can be easy to slip into a place of thinking that the dentist knows best, that the patient can't rely on his own good sense to make certain decisions about his care.

Part of what I gave up in practicing Same Day Dentistry is the mental comfort that comes with believing that you're the expert and you're the one in charge of the situation. When I gave up the idea of a full, planned-out schedule, I was stepping out and taking a leap of faith. And when I committed to the Same Day Dentistry concept, I also committed to getting out of my *physical* comfort zone.

That is, instead of hiding behind the safe façade of my office and my title, I venture out into the reception area to greet every patient. And I think this is where the patient truly begins to see me as someone with whom he, in turn, can be comfortable. I understand that I'm not in control of anything; I can't be in control of the patient's emotions, expectations, or finances. I can't be in control of whether or not he's going to come back for further work. All I can do is the best that I can do for him, to solve his problems *that day*. And I'm much better prepared to do that if I step out of that comfort zone and meet him where he is, as a human being, as a person who needs a compassionate advocate.

This can be a tough concept to get used to at first. It's scary. No matter how successful we are, no matter how many years of schooling and experience we've amassed, no matter how many awards and plaques line our office walls, we're no different than anyone else. Deep down, we want to be liked, and we hate rejection just as much as the next person.

But the real reward of stepping out of the comfort zone is success. Not just financial success—though I'm certain that will come if you're providing quality care and a compassionate experience for your patients—but *personal* success, as well. Nothing beats the feeling of being able to hold my head up high, knowing that I'm really making a difference in the lives of my patients. I wouldn't change the way I do business for anything—not a full schedule, not a Ferrari, and certainly not the conventional security of hiding in my office, away from the waiting room. And I'm willing to bet that if you're able to take a few slow, steady steps outside of your comfort zone, you're going to like the view out here too.

CHAPTER FOUR

The Same Day Triple Win:
Why Patients, Team, and Doctor All Do Better with Same Day Dentistry

Plenty of people love what they do, but that's not enough to keep them going in to the office day after day over the course of a long career. And plenty of professionals who provide a service love the people they provide that service to, but that's not enough to keep their payroll going and their accounts in the black. And there are plenty of wonderful customers and patients out there—especially when it comes to those seeking dentistry—who would love to find superior service from a trustworthy provider, but who either believe they can't afford it or don't believe it's out there.

Long ago, I never thought I'd come up with a solution that could address all these pain points. That pie-in-the-sky kind of thinking was for people with fewer student loans to worry about, I thought, or people without a family to support. I was happy (well, not exactly *happy*, but willing) to grind away in corporate dentistry and leave the big-picture thinking to other folks.

But I've always been the kind of person to reconsider and admit when I'm wrong. And I was more than happy to make just that sort of admission when I took the leap to start creating the Same Day Dentistry revolution. Because Same Day has something that no other model of dentistry has: the Same Day Triple Win.

If that sounds like an exciting proposition, that's because it is. Everything that we've talked about in the book so far—all of my motivation behind starting over in that modest strip-mall space and creating a different type of life and career for myself—can be encapsulated in that simple phrase.

Let's look at the Triple Win through the lens of a typical situation that we see in my office. A patient comes in; we'll call her "Sue." She hasn't been to the dentist in a while, and she's never been to our practice, but she found our location approachable and saw that we had good reviews. She was also intrigued by the idea of Same Day Dentistry. Being a working mom with more than a full schedule to deal with, she assumed that Same Day Dentistry might be the way to go if she were going to finally fit in taking care of her dental issues.

These days, it's hard enough for patients like Sue to prioritize *scheduled* dental cleanings and doctor's visits for themselves. Usually, working moms and dads put off their own care until the very last minute. But Sue's situation had already gone past last minute and well into dental emergency. She'd been meaning to make time to go to the dentist for a while. Toothaches here and there probably spelled cavities, she knew, but the night before her visit, she'd shattered a tooth. By the time she had gotten the kids off to school, arranged coverage at work, and rolled into the office, the pain was so severe that she was in tears. And her pain was compounded by every working parent's enemy: the ticking clock.

Even as she sat at my desk in visible pain, she tried to minimize her needs.

"Is there any way you can just patch it up?" she asked. "I don't think I have time for anything really complicated. I'll be fine if I can make it a little longer. I'll schedule an appointment for the next time I can take a day off."

I could see her mentally tallying when that "next time" might be. In the earlier days of my career, I had often made the mistake of thinking that patients like Sue didn't recognize good dental care when they saw it, or else didn't appreciate it or think it was important. Lacking the compassion of a more seasoned version of myself, I had assumed that they didn't know enough to understand what they needed. *I* was the dentist after all; why was *the patient* telling me that I needed to hurry up and give them some half-baked patch job?

But this was before Same Day Dentistry, and before I understood how false that assumption was. It wasn't as though Sue didn't care about her teeth. It was more that everyone else's needs came first. Her family needed her, her job needed her, and when she finally had time for herself (which she took only because she absolutely *had* to, when it was an emergency), she was worried about all the responsibilities piling up while she was sitting in our office. She was worried that she'd have to spend more time (and money) that she couldn't spare coming back to sit in the exam room again for follow-up visits, and worrying about all the work it would take to coordinate those visits around her children, her husband, and her job. I noticed, though, that when I started to explain the possibilities for treatment to her, she began to relax. Pleasantly surprised even through all that pain, she was starting to see beyond a patch job, a big bill, and a chunk of personal time away from the office. She could see the light at the end of the tunnel, the Triple Win clearly visible on the other side.

Some things have changed over the years. My view of patients has changed. My process has changed. My practice is growing, and my satisfaction with my career has never been higher. I've been able to do more of the kind of dentistry that I have always wanted to do, increase my quality, and increase my efficiency. But some things remain the same: several years into Same Day Dentistry, seeing the relief on a patient's face as I explain our process and how that patient will benefit from the Same Day Triple Win is every bit as rewarding today as it was on my first day in the office.

Winner #1: The Patient

The first (and my personal favorite) beneficiary of the Triple Win in this case is Sue. When she comes into the office with a broken tooth, instead of inundating her with a laundry list of costly procedures and issues to follow up on (or, for that matter, giving her a so-called "solution" that's just going to have her coming back in tears at some point in the near future), we can present an alternative. With the technology we have available, and with the team we've trained to assist, we can confidently tell Sue that she can get a crown made for her today.

"No rescheduling, no losing more work time," we can tell her. "We can take care of this today."

Financially, it may cost Sue a little more than a temporary fix would, but she'll more than make up for it with the time and agony she saves down the line, weeks or months or years from now, when she's out getting her to-do list tackled instead of sitting in my chair again. And because of our policy of transparency and consistency when it comes to our prices, which are listed plain as day on our website, that financial premium isn't going to be as surprising to Sue when we give her an estimate of what the procedure will cost. But I've found that when it comes to getting quality dental care done right the first time (and done right *quickly),* money is typically less important to patients than their trust and their time.

In fact, one of the pleasant surprises of Same Day Dentistry is that the patient will often end up taking advantage of *more* services rather than fewer. This is a fact that never ceases to impress my colleagues in the field. How often do you have patients looking to get *more* work done than what they originally came seeking? The Same Day Dentistry philosophy is anything but typical, even for the "typical" patient.

In Sue's case, for example, when we presented her with the crown solution to solve her immediate and most pressing complaint, we were able to present her with a menu of additional services that we could fit in just by virtue of the fact that we were expanding a one-hour "patch up" visit into a two- or two-and-a-half-hour crown procedure. There were other problem areas nearby that needed shoring up in order to ensure continued comfort and health for Sue. Because we had gained her trust with our transparency and our ability to tell her with confidence that her crown could be done in just one appointment, she was more than amenable to having adjacent work done at the same time. And at the end of her appointment, she was able to leave with a new crown, new fillings, and *none* of the pain and anxiety that she walked in with.

Sue was leaving with more money in her pocket, as well. Because of our streamlined process, including the modest-looking location that attracted her in the first place, we're able to pass along a good deal of savings. Because our productivity for the visit was increased and because we can take care of more during one visit rather than setting up additional appointments, which carry additional costs of time and space and materials, we don't have to charge for those extra visits. We don't have to factor into our cost the potential for missed appointments, and so neither does Sue.

And, let's not forget about her first priority: she was able to leave with plenty of time to pick up her kids from school.

Winner #2: The Team

While the happiness of patients like Sue will always represent a chief concern of mine, my team is right up there when it comes to people I want to keep smiling. Fortunately, the Same Day Dentistry philosophy makes that easier.

Continuing with the example of Sue's case, my team comes out on top too. And that's a very good thing, because this whole process wouldn't work without my team! The word "team" is particularly apt here; after all, around the office, we call our smooth Same Day Dentistry process "passing the ball." It's a pretty well-orchestrated system at this point, starting from when the patient calls in or is greeted, and flowing from there. Because my team is so involved with the coordination of care with the patient after I've interviewed him or her, there are no surprises for anyone. Everyone knows about how long the visit will take, and we can plan accordingly. My assistants are not diagnosing, but at this point, they're able to help the patient make some likely interpretations based on their charts and X-rays. They're as familiar and invested in the outcomes as I am.

This emphasis on efficiency and productivity is important to my team's happiness too. Because sometimes we're going to have to fit more patients in and stay past "quitting time" to get them all to a Same Day solution, we need to be as efficient as possible to keep things sustainable for everyone in our office.

Everyone does his or her part in that—from the dental assistant who helps the patient get comfortable and understand his or her problem, to the administrators who set up financial and insurance arrangements. I'm in there, too, obviously, doing the diagnosis and carrying out what the patient has decided upon in terms of his or her treatment plan. And throughout this process, efficiency stays at the front of our minds.

Take Sue's case: Instead of a one-hour patch job that would lead to other appointments down the line (possibly other *broken* appointments, if Sue was unsatisfied or unable to keep the return appointment she had booked), the team completed procedures that helped to triple our productivity in the same amount of time. And during that time, their directives had all been clear. No one has to focus on sales or the future, and no one has to take focus away from the patient to worry about the unknowns, like whether or not we'll have missed appointments down the line that will cost us time, money, and emotional frustration. Because we've been as productive as we possibly can be, and efficient as we possibly can be, that's all going to sort itself out pretty reliably.

But more than being productive, my team is winning when it comes to the fuzzy stuff: the honesty and pride they feel while working in such a transparent system. I love hearing my dental assistant Debbie talking to patients and proudly saying that, when the issue of cost comes up, she knows for a fact that our bottom line isn't artificially inflated.

"Doc doesn't have to worry about flying a big expensive airplane or anything like that," she'll say. "But he does have a really nice bicycle!"

The team knows that they can feel good about helping everyday people with what amounts to a significant expense. And they can feel this way because they're a part of making that solution. By helping to control costs through our efficient and transparent process, we're able to deliver more dentistry on time and on budget, stretching the clock and the dollar for the patient. On those long days when we've got to skip going straight home for dinner, or during those times when we're knee-deep in charts and phone calls and things to check off our lists, that's the kind of thing that keeps you going!

And speaking of finances, there's an important incentive for my staff built into the way we do things—another way they "win." The better the office does, the better *they* do. Our transparency trickles down to the staff in this way: We all know what our overhead is and we all watch the numbers. At the end of the month, if our collections exceed our overhead—which they usually do—profit sharing kicks in.

The better we perform, the better our collections are. My team members have had months where, after splitting our profits per our agreement, they've increased their base-pay income by over ten dollars an hour. But like our "ball passing," this doesn't work unless everyone is playing together and on a high level. Everyone needs to be willing to go that extra mile, and so the team has an incentive to encourage that cohesive bond and productive environment. This has the added benefit of self-regulation. On the rare occasion in which there has been a team member who wasn't pulling his or her weight, they can course correct. I've long learned not to underestimate the culture that results from common goals!

The transparency that we encourage in the profit-sharing system is entwined with the transparency that makes it possible for all members of our team to have a deep and innate understanding of how our sometimes swiftly changing Same Day schedule works. We check in with each other first thing every day and look at where our schedule might have some give. We're all equally invested in and educated on what's going on in the office, day in and day out. And our structure and transparency—this idea that I'm not just the man behind the curtain, pulling the strings, but rather, that our entire team is involved in balancing a dynamic schedule—gives everyone the power to weigh in on whether or not we can take an additional case late in the day. Making the Same Day Dentistry principles work is always an all-hands-on-deck-type enterprise, and all of those hands should get a vote.

I know that there are some dentists who would look at me a little askew if they knew that I am sharing the profits in a business in which I am the sole owner. But here's the thing: Even though I'm the sole owner, I'm far from being the sole team member. We're all a part of the success, and so we all should be party to the spoils of that success.

Now, we weren't able to do this from day one; it wasn't until about a year after we opened our practice and really got the hang of how this would all work that we could begin our profit-sharing system. But now, a couple of years into that system, I'm confident that it's an incentive that's ripe for replication, particularly in the Same Day Dentistry model.

Winner #3: The Dentist

Some would say I've saved the best for last, but you can probably tell that for me, taking care of number one doesn't come first. I don't want to overlook this point, though, because chances are, you've picked up this book because you're looking to make a change.

Maybe you're a young dentist at the start of your career, weighed down by splitting your time between different corporate-style offices just to make ends meet. Maybe you're nearing retirement age and hoping to leave a different kind of legacy for your junior dentists and your own loyal team members. Or maybe you're just like I was: in the prime of my career and coming to terms with the fact that things weren't quite working anymore.

Whatever the case may be, I love that I'm able to say with confidence that you'll win too when it comes to practicing the Same Day Dentistry model. Part of your winnings will come in the form of direct financial security and the professional benefits of having a thriving practice. But, if I know you (and I think I might!), a large part of your winnings won't be about you at all. The prizes will be those relieved smiles on the faces of patients who are no longer in pain. Or the trophies you'll collect in the form of poolside toasts with your staff members at an all-expenses-paid office trip.

Whatever the rewards end up being for you, they're sure to be great ones.

CHAPTER FIVE

What to Expect If You're a Same Day Dentistry Patient

A s dentists in our own domain, we have a certain level of comfort over any process or protocol. No matter if you've just turned your whole office upside down to go from "Someday" to "Same Day," you've at least got an idea of what to expect from the experience. But what about your patients?

I'm happy when my patients are happy. And I know that my patients are happiest when they are comfortable, both in and out of my chair. I know that this comes from trust, transparency, and an attention to detail that prizes the patient experience above all else. So it's with this in mind that I've designed the Same Day Dentistry experience, soup to nuts.

Clicking, Calling, and Coming By: Putting the Same Day Dentistry Mission out There from the Get-go

We've talked a bit already about how in today's times, there's a pretty good chance that patients will have checked out your practice online before ever setting foot in your office. That's what being a customer in the digital age is all about. With Yelp, Facebook, and Twitter, opinions and experiences are out there for everyone to see, for better or worse. For any business owner, the idea that your reputation can be made or destroyed in 140 characters or fewer is more than a little frightening.

But—*surprise!*—I encourage you to think about this digital reality a little differently and view it as an opportunity. While you might not be able to control exactly what your patients are typing, you are *absolutely* in control of the experience that they have. This is one of those chicken-or-the-egg things in life: If you make patients happy, they will express their happiness. If you have happy patients, this instantaneous online customer-feedback space can bring in more patients for you to make happy. As social media use has blossomed, I've had more and more initial conversations with patients that begin with them telling me about glowing reviews they've read online, sometimes on a friend's page or feed. This is music to my ears; the value of that third-party validation can't be overstated.

What's more, you can also control the accessibility and transparency of your online presence. For instance, we put all of our fees right there on our website. This means that potential patients don't have to do much digging to see what services we offer and how much those services might cost.

We extend that transparency and warmth the old-fashioned way too. From the moment our office staff members answer the phone, patients can expect clear information and quality service. It seems like such an obvious thing, but it's something that's often overlooked, whether you're dealing with the cable company or your healthcare provider. When you're a Same Day Dentistry patient, you can expect that your call—whether you're in the middle of an emergent dental situation or you're just looking for information on services and costs—will be answered by a friendly, dedicated, and knowledgeable team member who is empowered to help you.

Finally, our office is in a high-visibility, high-traffic location that encourages drop-in visits. This should be a hallmark of any Same Day Dentistry practice.

Welcome to Same Day Dentistry: In the Waiting Room

They've read the reviews. They've made the call. Now it's time for the patient to pay us a visit.

My choice of the word "visit" isn't accidental. Unlike the typical dental office, where there might be a receptionist and a water cooler squeezed into a small, dimly lit room with a few uncomfortable chairs and outdated magazines, the experience of coming into our office is designed to feel more akin to sitting down in someone's living room. Partially owing to our choice of an affordable location, we've been able to invest in a large, bright, open space with multiple seating areas and desks, so that my team and I can easily migrate from patient to patient, literally *meeting them where they are.*

Whereas the first time a patient will typically interact with a dentist is pretty stressful and unbalanced—the dentist is standing while the patient is reclining in the chair, usually having already been bibbed and poked at by the hygienist or dental assistant— the Same Day Dentistry experience is designed to begin more like a casual conversation. Instead of meeting in an exam room, I greet patients in our waiting room and then, when they are ready, move with them to my desk.

Getting to Know You: The First Conversation

This initial conversation is just as much about the patient getting to know me as it is about me getting to know the patient. This doesn't mean that I'm the one doing the talking; this isn't about me, and it's not my story that anyone should be interested in. The fact that I'm asking the patients to tell me *their* story, to tell me about what they want to have done today, that speaks volumes about my personality, my compassion, and my interest in them both as patients and *as people*.

After the initial "What brings you in here today?" or "How can I help you?" I might ask the patient about how he or she found us, what his or her past experiences with dentistry have been, and so forth. There's no cookie-cutter approach to the interview process; instead, it's all about truly *listening* and responding appropriately. It's about digging deeper, but with a gentle and empathic touch. Sometimes, for example, I'll have a patient who is absolutely terrified of the dentist. I want to get to the root of that problem. What has traumatized him or her about past experiences? What could have been done to make those experiences better? By hearing each patient out at the beginning of each visit, I know he or she will be significantly more at ease when it's time for us to meet when he or she is in a more vulnerable position in the exam room.

This doesn't have to take too much time or energy, either. I genuinely like interacting with my patients, as I'm sure most of my fellow dentists do, as well. But we're only human, and we have limitations: a packed schedule, an intertwined staff that heavily relies on the efficiency of everyone on the team from the top down, etc. The interview process, while high-touch and thorough, doesn't have to take a lot of time. It truly depends on the individual; it could take two minutes or it could take five. The bottom line is that this is time well spent if you spend it wisely. If you truly listen, if you focus, and if you put the patient at ease, your investment will pay dividends. Every time I have a patient say something like, "I've never had a doctor come and talk to me like this before," I know that this initial contact has gone a long way to breaking down those barriers and building up their trust level.

Passing the Ball: The Team Takes Its Queue

There's an important difference between passing the ball and passing the buck. In my team environment, we often talk about "passing the ball"—in this case, moving the patient from person to person and throughout the Same Day process in the most efficient manner possible. After I've spent time developing a relationship with the patient and getting the big picture of his

also get a sense of what it is the patient is leaning toward doing as we sort out priorities and I provide my professional opinion.

Costs, Decisions, Treatment: Making a Plan for Same Day Dentistry Solutions

When the exam is over and the patient is ready to make his or her decisions, there's still one piece of information left: the cost of the day's solutions.

Again, I always strive for clarity. And that's why I let the professionals take over—in this case, Terran, my front-desk manager. After hearing my assessment and getting to talk over his or her concerns, the patient then sits with Terran and the hygienist/assistant to make final determinations about what care will be taking place that day. Terran goes over the exact cost of care, so that there are no surprises about whatever course of action the patient chooses. If the patient insurance, we'll work to figure out what his or her financial responsibility will be. If the patient doesn't have insurance, we'll break down our prices. And since our patients have been free to compare costs using our website before coming into the office, they can be pretty confident that they're getting a good deal.

By the time I return, I'm ready to play the role that my staff lovingly refers to as "Dr. Bobblehead," meaning that whatever the treatment plan the patient feels comfortable with for that day, I'm going to nod my head and get started.

I know that some dentists will balk at the idea that they will not be present for the explanation of costs, citing the fact that many patients will object to procedures or hesitate, saying they need to go home and talk it over with their spouse, or they need to think about it more, or they're suddenly not in that much pain. "How will you make the sale!?" those dentists worry.

My response is that I don't have to worry about making the sale, primarily because of the comfort level and the approachable range of same-day services that we offer. Because I'm not trying to sell the patient on a months-long course of treatment, he or she can view each issue in a manageable, separate chunk. And no doubt because of the comfort and trust that the patient has built up with me and my team during the course of the appointment, that quality care is worth it to him or her.

That's an integral part of the beauty of Same Day Dentistry. If you can give your patients a solution *and do it today,* you're really helping them out. They're getting it done. Even with the patients whose anxiety is at an all-time high, at least you're always able to say, "We're going to be able to fix your (broken tooth, cavity, cracked filling, whatever the case might be) today. I know that you'd rather not do this. I know you'd rather be doing a million things instead of spending your afternoon here in my chair. But in two hours, it'll be over and done with. You'll be able to sleep tonight without pain. And you won't have to worry about coming back to get more useless temporary filler thrown onto that patch job."

I also don't want to have to worry about making the sale because *it's not up to me to be a salesman.* Instead, it's up to me to be an advocate and educator for my patients. At the point when they're making game-time decisions about whether or not they can pay for a certain procedure on a certain day, I've given them all the information. I've given them my time. I've given them all I've got—outside of my services, of course. This, as a dentist, is what I have to give. I don't have salesmanship or gamesmanship. If I did, I'd be in a different industry. And I think my patients appreciate that I've chosen the path that I've chosen, because I don't know many people who would want to see a salesman for their dental care, just like you wouldn't want to try to buy a car from a dentist!

No Credit, No Problem: We Don't Take It Anyway

Although I used to accept credit (such as the popular health-care brand CareCredit) earlier on in my practice, I have made it a policy at Same Day Dental to do away with any credit, installment plans, or billing. This doesn't mean that we're a high-end-only practice; most of our patients are working people, just like you and me. And this doesn't mean we're unaffordable.

Actually, the fact that we don't take credit means *exactly the opposite*. It means that we don't have to worry about tacking on service fees to cover our costs of dealing with the credit companies or inflating our prices across the board to make up for revenue lost to collections. It means that we don't have to spend valuable time haggling with customers and credit companies over the phone. It means there's no middleman when it comes to patient care. And, most of all, it aligns with our objective to squash the idea that money is the main objective of quality dentistry.

The dental-credit industry is built on the idea that getting patients to take on a payment plan is going to be the only way that they'll fork over the cash for a quality procedure. This is a self-fulfilling prophecy. If we go into our work with the defeatist attitude that we're: 1) unable to offer patients the services they need at a price they can afford, and 2) unable to provide services that live up to their value, then we might as well quit before we get started and save ourselves all some time and grief!

It's true that some patients have so many issues to address that their entire course of care is unaffordable. But by keeping our costs low and our options flexible, we're still able to work with those patients. Instead of pushing them to sign up for credit that they ultimately can't pay back, why not work to find a schedule that works for their time, their finances, *and* their health? If a patient has to split up care over several appointments, we're there for them. If he or she has the finances to get the work done right away and it's urgent enough, we're there to make that happen too.

And one more thing: My bottom line isn't the bottom line. It's my patients. I'd never be so worried about making payroll that I would push a patient to sign up for an installment plan for work he or she couldn't afford in the first place. I've arranged my practice so that I'm fortunate enough that we have our operating costs covered without taking a personal toll on our patients to make that number.

At Same Day Dentistry, Patient Comfort Is a Right, Not an Option

At the end of the day, when you strip away all of the philosophical tenets that led me to building a more comfortable business environment for myself and my staff, in which we could grow and sustainably practice the kind of dentistry we wanted, you're left with nothing to focus on but patient comfort. This is what I love about the Same Day Dentistry practice we've built. Ultimately, *comfort* is what I want patients to expect when they sign up to be a Same Day Dentistry patient.

That desire has shaped how I've designed everything in this practice. From our waiting area to the painless X-rays in our first patient visit to the efficient procedures that are meant to minimize time and discomfort in the dental chair, I want the patient's comfort to be a right, not an optional luxury.

I can't emphasize this enough. We humans are sensitive when vulnerable, and our mouths are among our most sensitive, intimate areas. My staff and I do not take for granted that patients who come to us seeking care—many of whom we are meeting for the very first time—have given us permission to enter and treat this intimate part of their body. We do not take this responsibility lightly. Instead, we commit ourselves to doing our very best to ensure the comfort of those patients, to make sure they feel taken care of, as well as healed, during their time of vulnerability and pain. We believe it is truly an honor to be trusted in this way by people who were strangers when they walked into our office. We are so thankful to be chosen by them, and we look forward to ensuring comfort and care for many years to come.

Here are just a few of the amazing patient reviews that our practice has collected over the years of helping our community find comfortable, quality Same Day Dentistry care!

"I am very pleased with my treatment. Dr. Cole and staff were pleasant, professional and helpful. They explored all my treatment options and how the choices would affect my dental health. They were thorough in explaining my treatment and cost of treatment. They gave me a precise outline of what treatment cost and what insurance would cover and what I was responsible for paying myself before we started the procedure. I most definitely will be visiting their office for my future dental needs."

—Amy C., July 2016

"I've been coming here for a few years. Always have a pleasant experience! State of the art technology with friendly staff and a doctor that noticeably loves his job and cares about the comfort of his patients."

—Lee P., May 2016

"I had the BEST EXPERIENCE at this dental clinic the entire staff was awesome! I'm the type of person who is painfully afraid and everyone was totally compassionate."

—Anonymous, April 2016

"Dr. Cole is a remarkably, caring, knowledgeable, compassionate dentist. I have had nothing but a top notch experience every time."

—Lisa G., December 2015

CHAPTER SIX

Location, Location, Location
*Can You Really Practice Dentistry
in a Strip Mall?*

"If you build it, they will come."

Most of you will recognize this quote as the apocryphal advice whispered to Kevin Costner's character among the waving stalks of corn in *Field of Dreams*. I know, I know, they were talking about a baseball field, but I like to think of it as applying equally to Same Day Dentistry!

One of the premises behind my Same Day Dentistry philosophy is that if you build a quality dental practice, patients will come, no matter if it looks or feels like what they expect of a typical dental office. If you build the right dental practice for yourself, you and your team (the *right* team) will find happiness there too. There is no one-size-fits-all way to do this. I wanted to preface this chapter with this note so that you will keep it in mind as you're reading. If something sounds like it really won't work for you, you're free to disregard it. But if it sounds like something you might be open to, I encourage you to shed your preconceived notions about what's right and what's possible, and stick, instead, to what's *true for you*.

Because if you build it (it, being a high-quality dental practice), they *will* come. Even if you're tucked into a commercial strip mall next to a dry cleaner and a nail salon.

Location, Location, Location

What I'm about to say might sound a tad contradictory, given my affinity for the famous advice from *Field of Dreams,* but bear with me and keep in mind that sometimes our preconceptions are what hold us back. What you find just might surprise you.

I never was one to believe in that old real estate adage, "location, location, location" as much as I do now that I'm three years into my current practice. I thought, somewhat naïvely I suppose, that the *Field of Dreams* advice meant that patients would find me *regardless* of location. In fact, this wasn't the case. It wasn't the case when I was tucked into the far southwest corner of a faceless medical complex or on the third floor of a professional building, my practice buried among the names of many other medical and dental professionals. To get patients to come to *those* locations —locations that I felt represented the "right" place for a dentist to be—I was spending a large amount of money and effort to advertise my services, with minimal impact.

Contrast this with my current location, which has clear signage and a lot of commercial and road traffic, and the wiser choice is clear.

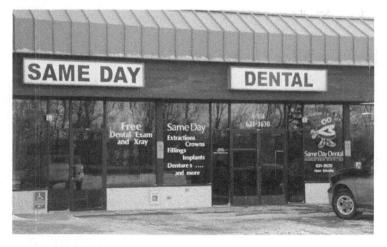

Whereas before, I would only have patients coming in for prearranged appointments, or patients who knew about us through our advertising, I regularly notice that our foot traffic has increased now that we're in our current location. I see people slowing down for the speed bump in the parking lot and craning their necks to check us out. *"Is there really a dentist right by my dry cleaner?"*

This kind of exposure is a boon to any practice, but it's absolutely essential to a Same Day Dentistry practice, which makes a good portion of its revenue by encouraging walk-in and emergency appointments. I'll also hear from patients that our location was ultimately what made them feel comfortable approaching us. One day, after running errands in the area a few times and seeing our open, conveniently located space, they found the courage to stop putting off their dental health and walk on in. And when new patients who *haven't* seen us in person call and ask where we're located, it's very easy to give them directions, particularly in small-town Alaska: we're right there next to the IHOP, or right around the corner from Jo-Ann Fabrics!

Hearing from patients that our ease of access was one of the factors that drove their decision to spend their hard-earned dollars and scarce time with us has been incredibly rewarding for me, especially when I consider the trepidation that I once had before making this leap into my current practice. I, like many of my peers, had this preconception, this sort of "ivory tower" complex. And given all the time and money I spent on my training, I can't really blame my younger, more anxious self. But part of this journey has been about getting to know my true self. And the truth is? That self is more comfortable in this new professional home.

The location hasn't just attracted patients, either. I've spoken at length already about how important it is that the team in a Same Day Dentistry practice shares the vision and down-to-earth qualities that I've espoused within these pages. In the case of Ashley, one of our front-desk representatives, the location of our office was what brought her into the Same Day Dentistry family. Like many of our patients, she was initially surprised by our location, but like those same patients, this approachability came to be a part of what she loved about our office.

I admire that Ashley was able to be honest with me about her thoughts because it's given me insight into what our patient experience might be like. And I want to share them with you just as plainly and honestly so that you might see how this would translate to your own patients, as well as your Same Day Dentistry team.

My Same Day Dentistry Story — Ashley

"I had been in the shopping plaza a few times before, and noticed that there was a dental practice mixed in with the shops. I didn't know what to think. I'd never seen a dental office in a location like this, right next to a Chinese restaurant. Was it actually going to be part of the same business? Was this just a signage mix-up? I wasn't sure.

But when I went in to drop off my resume, I saw that not only was I definitely in a clean, professional dental office, but I was also in exactly the kind of office that I would want to work in. The space radiated friendliness and openness. It was a no-frills approach without any walls up—literally or figuratively. I'm definitely in the right place, I thought."

Ashley isn't alone in her opinion. I've had many patients comment along the same lines upon seeing our transparent, down-to-earth approach from the get-go. A lot of that can be attributed to the psychological effect of having a large, open reception area where truly nonthreatening patient–dentist conversations can be held. In the typical dental setting, the price per square foot of real estate is so high that you can't afford to leave so much of it open and free-flowing. But because I was willing to think outside the box and choose a location that not many would have considered, I was gifted with this spacious, brilliant surprise.

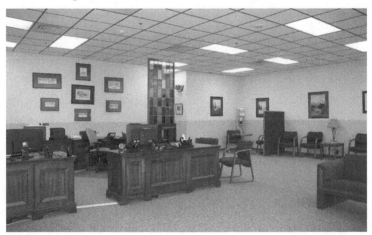

Daring to Dream

When we started in our 2,800-square-foot space, we were only using half of it. At the time, I couldn't imagine that we'd use more; I thought that we could use the rest for storage, or add a break room. This was the downtrodden Charlie talking; I had gotten into the mentality that "good enough" was, well, good enough!

But another side effect of having a big space has been that we've been able to fill that space with equally big dreams. When I had a losing mentality—or, if I'm being generous, a "good enough" mentality—it was easy to discount the possibilities of the extra space we had. But as time went on and we expanded, I was so thankful that we had the room to grow. And I noticed that the bigger I dreamed, the bigger we were able to get. I let myself think beyond the historical expectations that I'd locked myself into from years of working in typical corporate dental offices. And, like the feeling of satisfaction I got when I was on the beach with my staff in Turks and Caicos, it doesn't get much better than surveying all that Same Day Dental has become in response to daring to dream. Three years in, and we've got seven dental chairs where we used to have only three. We just brought on an associate dentist. And we're still going—and *growing*—strong.

Neighbors and Community

I have to admit, I haven't talked to many dentists about what they think about our location. Part of this shift in my career and my practice has been about staying true to my own values, and not measuring myself against others. But I've been a dentist long enough to know how the "typical" dentist might think, and that includes understanding why there might be some resistance to the idea of a location with a greater community feel.

By nature, dentists are technicians. We are trained to be impressed by the high-tech, the high-end. We're naturally inclined to want the top-of-the-line technology, to be attracted to the brand-name products. And we feel this way, in part, because we've associated this as being better for our patients. We get trapped into thinking that the clothes make the man, so to speak, that the best dental chair on the market, or the best drill, will make us the best dentist we can be.

Make no mistake, I'm not downplaying the importance of quality equipment. I'm not saying that professionals shouldn't be up to date on the latest technology and trends (I touted the benefits of my all-digital arsenal in the last chapter, after all!). But there's no sense in thinking that this is any substitute for high-quality *care*. The patients don't understand high-tech on the level that we do, but they do *feel* the benefits of a high-touch relationship. They see and understand a nonthreatening environment.

I would challenge you, as I challenged myself in the beginning of this process, to truly, honestly assess what it is about the nature of high-gloss, high-status spaces that puts you at ease. Is it really that you think you are doing the best you can for your patients, or is it that you're compensating for your own insecurities? Just speaking for myself, I know that I was hiding behind a location that I felt was befitting of a dentist. And again, speaking for myself, I know that now, in my current location, I've reaped the rewards of being true to myself, which have included a higher sense of authenticity and connection with my community.

Part of that is literal. Because I am within a community of merchants, I am part of a thriving commercial center that operates on some level like its own neighborhood. Not only are the customers of these businesses also customers of my business, but the hardworking men and women who keep the dry cleaner, the IHOP, the Chinese restaurant next door, and the nail salon a few doors down running day in and day out are also people I'm lucky enough to count among my patients.

Another way I benefit from the patterns and traffic of my neighboring businesses is that they provide goods and services beyond the 9-to-5, Monday-to-Friday sphere. Some of these retailers are open on Saturdays—others, on Sundays— and some keep late hours, often until nine o'clock at night. This contributes to a bustling commercial center that attracts customers with confidence at all hours, which is meaningful to many of *our* customers seeking Same Day Dentistry services on their off time, so as not to eat into their workdays. My location has truly helped me to meet my customers where they are. If you build it, they will come . . . if they can find you.

I wish that I could claim to be smart enough to have anticipated that this would be the case; I can't tell you that in good conscience, but one can dream! Instead, it was more of a serendipitous occurrence; I needed a space, and this space was available. I was at a point in my career when I was facing a formidable transition. I didn't have a lot of time, money, or other resources—but what I did have was the possibility of this space. And because I was a little bit down on my luck and was forcing myself to leave my comfort zone and get creative, I allowed myself to be open to something that I wouldn't normally have even considered. And my life has been so much better for it—not to mention my profit margins, which have only grown as a result of my location and which are significantly less weighed down by the fixed cost of a high-rent office in a more "traditional" location.

We all know the old saying about lemons and lemonade, and being truly thirsty can help drive that all the more.

Final Thoughts on Location

I think you know me well enough now to know that I'm not going to try to sell you a formula. I'm not going to say that if you do "steps one through ten," you can build a Same Day Dentistry model that works for you. But what I *will* say is that it's possible to find something that really *does* work for you if you're willing to listen to your most true self.

I don't, by any means. have this all figured out; life is a life-long process by nature. But I do have a few ideas that you're welcome to take and adapt to your own life, your own truth.

- Be genuine in all things. Location is no exception. If you want to serve a particular community, and really be a part of that community, *go to where that community is.* Set up shop there. Don't feel like you have to hang your shingle in the fanciest part of town just because it will give you a good reputation. It won't; it'll just give you a big rent bill each month.

- Don't fall victim to advertisements. This is true of real estate ads, and it's true of less obvious "ads": the pictures and profiles in the journals of our profession. Just because something works for one dentist doesn't mean it will work for you. Just because someone has paid thousands of dollars for ad placement doesn't mean that his or her product or style is any better than yours.

- Surround yourself by an office staff that supports who you truly are.
- Don't underestimate the value of foot traffic. Does your potential location have other retailers nearby? Is there a sidewalk? Is it easy to access for those without cars? Is it near public transportation? Is it near an intersection, giving drivers time to see your signage?
- Go with your gut. Be where you want to be. Your work can't be everything, or your work will suffer along with your life. I found my true north in Alaska; yours might be in the middle of the country. Wherever it is, it's yours to find and yours to thrive in.

CHAPTER SEVEN

Passing the Savings Along to the Patient

The Economics of Same Day Dentistry

When it comes to running a business, even a novice knows that he or she must have a handle on two directions of cash flow: in and out. Once the fixed costs are known, these must be balanced against income projections and then, hopefully, if all goes well, profit projections. After looking at all the data, a savvy businessperson will decide what profit percentage he or she would like to strive for, and then move operations forward on that basis.

We dentists, though, aren't first and foremost businesspeople. We're providers of dental care. I can't speak for everyone, but I think that very reasoning is what you'll find when you get down to the bottom of any dentist's business model. It doesn't matter how good you are at dentistry; business is still a struggle for many of us.

Because of this, I've found it far more common for dentists to look to external sources for validation rather than making projections and goals based on their own needs and desires. Instead of thinking about what makes the most sense for them, these dentists will look to see what their peers are charging for certain services, and then try to make comparable offerings, regardless of whether this makes sense for *their* needs and *their* expenses. Or, just as commonly, dentists will find out what insurance will reimburse them for, and then bump up the ceiling of their services accordingly to increase their profit margins. This benefits neither the dentist nor the patient in the end: the patient usually has to stretch to afford the service, and the dentist is relegating far too much power to external factors such as the fickle reimbursement policies of insurance companies.

This was part of what I wanted to escape when I started Same Day Dentistry. I wanted to take a more specific approach to my practice—not just because I wanted to practice the way that I wanted to practice, but because I knew that I could set up an economic model that would benefit both my practice *and* my patients. Instead of sticking with the typical corporate model, I've taken the approach of being more specific about knowing what my costs are, arranging for a fair profit, and then designing my fees per service based upon what we need to generate per hour per operating room to meet our expenses and generate the profit level that works for us.

And how does that trickle down to the patient? It depends on the individual situation, of course, but I can tell you this: in my market, where I practice, I've been able to offer dental services around 20 percent to 30 percent *below* the cost of my peers. That's been music to my patients' ears.

Why Go Lower?

I don't blame you if you're wondering, *What's the point in going lower? If you have that much room between what you're charging and what your peers are charging, where's the harm in closing that gap a little bit? You'll still have a competitive advantage.*

That might be what makes the most sense for you—and I mean this in the most nonjudgmental way possible. Make no mistake: Same Day Dentistry, and the particular way in which I practice it, is a method. It is by no means a formula. There's nowhere in this book where I will tell you that in order to find your way to a successful Same Day Dentistry practice, you'll need to do X, Y, and Z. It simply doesn't work like that.

With that caveat, I can explain more about why I charge what I charge and how I'm able to do so. It's about sustainability for the patients, first and foremost. While I've spoken at length about addressing obstacles other than cost (quality, for example), cost is still an obstacle for many of my patients. I've put in the time with the numbers, and what I've arrived at is a schedule of fees that make sense for my practice, while at the same time, ensuring that much of the care we offer is affordable to much of our clientele.

It's important for me to treat everyone equally: I want the cash patient to receive the same care as a patient with premium insurance coverage, and I want the patient with premium insurance coverage to get the same care that a Medicaid patient will receive. I don't extend credit and I don't have a sliding scale that's higher for patients who can afford to pay more than others.

Some would criticize me for leaving money on the table, particularly where the patients with ample insurance coverage are concerned. "Why," they ask, "would you not charge a higher fee for insurance, knowing that the insurance company will pay more for the service?"

The answer is twofold: one, because I know that I can operate without that fabricated cushion, and two, because I know that most of my patients will still have out-of-pocket expenses even if they *do* have coverage. And charging less overall may translate to patients taking advantage of more services and procedures because they can afford to do so.

The goodwill that this kind of transparency and affordability engender will often result in a snowball effect. Take, for example, a recent patient I had who came in to our office after he found our fees posted on our website. He had a dentist he had been going to see regularly for years, but the cost comparison between his regular dentist and Same Day Dental gave him pause. He wanted to see what we were all about. Because he liked what he saw, he eventually brought his whole family to the practice. For price-sensitive patients, the transparency of pricing and the lower costs act as a draw. He came for the good deal, and he stayed for the service. Could I have charged more for his visit than I did and come out even further ahead on my profits for the visit? Yes. Would he have brought his entire family over to my practice when they were otherwise happy with their existing dentist? No. The multiplier of a satisfied customer was huge in this case.

Some of our cost savings end up being a boon to our patients because of concerns that are specific to practicing dentistry in

Alaska, where it's common to see individuals living in areas only accessible by airplane or ferry. One such patient—I'll call her "Marcy"—had to come in recently by airplane on a weekend, something that our flexible hours made possible. For Marcy, flying in solely for a dental appointment is a significant drain on finances as well as the valuable resource of time. In her case, we need to make not only the *cost* of the visit work for her, but the logistics of the visit—particularly the time it takes to complete the procedure—work as well. By following our ethics of efficiency that I've outlined earlier in this book, we are able to save Marcy the substantial cost and time of follow-up visits.

But not only does this kind of practice save the patient money; it saves the office significant overhead costs. We know, for example, that using the technology we've invested in, we can complete a crown in one same-day visit as opposed to stretching the procedure over two days. By not having to set up and break down the dental operatory each time, we slash further into that overhead. We save an hour of chair time. We save on the laboratory fees. We also save the patient—and ourselves—frustration, time, and money with problems that can arise between visits on a two-visit procedure.

Why Same Day Dentistry Means Fewer Cancellations

Another important component of our economic model is that by completing these procedures in the same day, we're decreasing the probability of missed, canceled, or rescheduled appointments across the board. That's a boon to both patient and provider, and we can pass those savings along to the patient, as well.

In life, emergencies happen; no one, no matter how considerate or well organized he or she is, can say he or she has *never* had to cancel or reschedule an appointment at the last minute. I certainly can't make that claim. I want to say up front that we absolutely understand that emergencies happen: people get sick, cars break down, and worse. But because with Same Day Dentistry, more patients are getting more work done in one visit than if it were spread across several, there are fewer opportunities for those emergencies to occur. They're already in the chair, after all.

There are patients who appear to take cancellation for granted, canceling with little or no notice when the whim strikes them. *He's got enough to do,* they might think as they decide to stay in bed a little longer that morning. *He's not going to miss my appointment. It will give him some time to catch up on other things, even!*

*A*ny dentist will tell you, this is far from the case. Just speaking for my own practice, office production suffers by around $500 for each hour of the schedule that goes unused. I know this because I've made sure that I know what my cost breakdown is on a very specific level, as I noted earlier in the chapter. And that money doesn't all go to me; it's money that's being taken away from my dental assistant, my front-desk staff, my dental suppliers, my lease fund, and so on. It's lost revenue that can't be regained if I don't have someone waiting in the wings who is willing and able to take the slot.

Although since instituting the Same Day Dentistry methodology I've noticed a significant decline in missed and canceled appointments, I will occasionally have patients who have a scheduled appointment and do not cancel within the required timeframe. Sometimes, these patients have good reasons—and sometimes, they don't. Our office has instituted a "one strike" policy with such patients, meaning that if they miss a scheduled appointment without canceling far enough in advance and without a valid emergent excuse, they lose the chance to book appointments in advance. We'll never—and I mean *never*—turn away a patient who comes to see us on a walk-in basis. Those patients who have gotten that one strike and still come in for emergency care can attest to that. But I'm happy to report that by being up front about our expectations and our office's culture of mutual respect, we haven't had to give out many of those "one strike" violations.

Although I don't want to continue to play into the idea that everyone is terrified of the dentist, I do have patients who are more reluctant than average when it comes to visiting the dentist. Whether their anxiety springs from a negative prior experience or from their own fears, that anxiety is very real for them. One of the benefits of the Same Day Dentistry experience is that those patients in particular are less likely to cancel and miss appointments; their experience, when appropriate, is compressed into a same-day procedure, which ultimately makes going to the dentist feel more manageable. Not being faced with an overwhelming treatment plan that brings them back several times allows them to immediately cross off a significant item on their list of concerns.

I've heralded the importance of efficiency time and again throughout our journey together, and it's no different when it comes to cash flow. Having control of our cash flow is essential to understanding what our expenses and profits are, and how we can expect those to flow in and out of the business. This knowledge enables us to function in a smooth and sustainable manner.

It's no different for our patients on an individual level when it comes to payment. They need to plan their budget, and they need to know what to expect when it comes to affording the quality dental care we offer at Same Day Dental. To that end, I've instituted what I like to think about as a "no-surprise policy"—specifically, there are no surprises for the patient upon check-in, and no surprises for the patient upon checkout. Patients are given clear options as to treatment plans and the costs attached to those plans, and they agree to services accordingly based on those figures. In the case of patients who have insurance, our clear and simple accounting methodology has given us a very good idea of what each procedure will cost and what will be covered by insurance, enabling us to give the patient an accurate estimate of what their responsibility will be. Occasionally, a patient will walk away at that point, or ask to be rescheduled for a time in the future, when he can better afford the care. But when all is said and done, if a patient really wants or needs a particular service, he will find room in his budget for that service. If a patient is still not ready, we don't push him.

Why I'm So Comfortable Being So Transparent

It's entirely possible that you're reading this and looking at the pages—and by extension, me—a little askew. *So I get why you don't feel comfortable upping your charges to insurance,* you might be thinking, *but isn't it a little dangerous to be so transparent? Aren't you painting yourself into a corner when it comes to your pricing and your methodology?*

I've been in that place before, and I understand it well. In my case, the attitude was coming from a very defensive place. I felt that patients and passersby alike were making assumptions about me based on my profession, and so I felt that the less I shared about myself and my process, the better. I've always been self-conscious, always more sensitive than most, and so it's hard for me to hear throwaway comments about how rich all dentists must be and how we're criminals for charging what we do. I've bragged to you before about my very nice bike.

Once, when I was in the parking lot, I had a patient give me a friendly elbow and say, "Nice car, Dr. C. Is that yours?"

It wasn't, I told him. It was my hygienist's. Even then, he kept up with the ribbing.

"You're paying her too much, then!"

I've never been in the business of purely high-end dentistry. I've never tried to squeeze my patients for more than what our services were worth. My transparency is good for my patients, but selfishly, it's great for me; it's great for that defensive, sensitive guy who worries about what people think of his motives. I can hold my head high as I walk into work each day knowing that I'm helping people, and that I've got nothing to hide.

CHAPTER EIGHT

Why Same Day Dentistry Beats Corporate Dentistry Any Day

A n old saying dictates that you shouldn't judge a man until you've walked a mile in his shoes. While I want to be clear that this book shouldn't be construed as a judgment or an indictment of any sort—everyone has the right to do what makes him or her happiest in the way that fits him or her best—I do think that I can offer a point of view that encompasses both sides of this issue as far as dentistry is concerned.

What Do I Mean by "Corporate," Anyway?

To be fair, I want to address the fact that I'm speaking in generalities in this chapter. I would need to write another book to get into the specifics of all the different types of corporate dentistry programs that are out there! Suffice it to say, a corporate program is typically something you'd find promoted by a self-styled dental "guru" or consultant, one that can be easily replicated, with the dentist being a relatively disposable part of the entire proposition.

The first thing that you need to understand about corporate dentistry is that when you sign up to work in a corporate dental environment, **you are giving up ownership, autonomy, and control.** Just like a corporate environment in any trade, corporate dentistry is governed by higher policies written not by the dentists in the exam rooms themselves, but by health-care, legal, and HR generalists, sometimes with a dentist advisor somewhere in the mix.

Also, just as in other corporate environments, the sales and managerial staff are the driving force behind the business. As a dentist, this never sat well with me; the idea that *I* was the disposable part of a dental practice. I was the one who had trained in my field for years. I was the one who had put in the work. So why should I be the one left out in the cold when it came to decision making? After a while, I realized it was nothing personal, but rather, simply the way that corporate dentistry is constructed.

Corporate dentistry is designed to maximize the importance of communication skills in the sales force while minimizing the importance of communication skills for the dentist. The pressure on the dentist becomes subsumed by the pressure of the sales force: to boost the bottom line by focusing on selling hefty elective procedures and expensive treatment plans, often financed at exorbitant interest rates by credit programs. This is not to say that elective procedures, like Invisalign˚ and whitening, don't have their value to patients, or that there aren't situations in which comprehensive treatment plans are absolutely necessary for the patient's health and well-being. Indeed, there are always exceptions to the rule. But on the whole, subscribing to these practices as required by corporate dentistry is antithetical to the philosophy of putting the patient first.

It's one thing to have sales goals if you're a salesperson; it's quite another to have those goals if your job is to provide dental care to patients. It doesn't take much elaboration to show where the line might easily be crossed inappropriately. In corporate dentistry, there's such an emphasis on constructing elaborate treatment plans, and such pressure to upsell the patients, all without really addressing what the patient needs done that day. From the patient side, I'd imagine getting shuffled through the process at a corporate dental office—exams and X-rays followed by a laundry list of expensive procedures that they're being pressured to sign on for—can feel more like being in a used-car lot than the office of a health-care provider. And oftentimes, it's all for naught, because the patients are so turned off by that experience (not to mention those who are completely unable to afford the proposed treatment plan), they might not keep their follow-up appointments, resulting in lost revenue in the end for the dental office.

And speaking of salesmanship, I don't know about you, but I take pride in my work and in my knowledge of my craft. That hadn't been the case for me when I was working in a group practice (not exactly corporate dentistry, but much of the same abdication of control). I felt like my skills as a dentist were an afterthought, and I was encouraged to focus always on selling. And while I consider myself a very good dentist, I absolutely *don't* consider myself a good salesman. Instead of being happy to go to work each day, I came in already feeling defeated. I didn't know how to close a sale. I didn't get positive feedback on the numbers I was generating. And over and over again, that's what I was hearing from the top of the chain. Not compliments on my skills as a dentist, not "Great work, Dr. C.! You really helped that patient out today." Instead, I felt constantly on the chopping block—probably not unlike those salesmen at the used-car lot I mentioned earlier. And, as you'll remember from earlier in this book, I was eventually not just on the chopping block, but also *chopped*.

So, If It's So Bad, Why Do So Many Do It?

I am absolutely sympathetic to the plight of the dentist who finds himself grinding it out in a corporate environment, day in and day out, to little satisfaction. Corporate dentistry seems the only way to go when it comes to finding security, stability, and any hope of paying off what can be quite exorbitant school loans for all of our training. You're clocking in and clocking out, giving up freedom and control for what seems like a more consistent paycheck and, potentially, a retirement package.

For some dentists, that might work, especially if they're just out of dental school and the cost of opening up an office is prohibitive. Another attractive feature of corporate dentistry—at least, on its face—is that dentists entering a corporate environment for the first time can feel as though they can focus just on the dentistry, rather than on all of the unpleasant front-of-office stuff (sales, insurance, OSHA, etc.) that they'd rather not deal with. I've already debunked the sales issue; when the bottom line is what everyone is focused on, you're going to find yourself part of a sales team whether you like it or not, whether you meant to or not. And putting aside for a moment the ethics of treating a patient more like a sales goal than a patient, there's also the issue of where the profits are actually going. In the corporate model, those profit margins go straight to the corporation, *not* to the individual dentist. So at some point, if you're thinking that you should be sticking with corporate dentistry for financial gain, but you're not *seeing* any of that financial gain, well, by that metric, it's just not worth it.

There is no right or wrong answer to how to live one's life, other than to live it authentically (and that's still a work in progress for me, make no mistake). But for those who got into the field because they wanted to be a sole proprietor, to be their own boss, and to see their business grow over time, the corporate path is not the one to take—at least not when you have a choice to walk a different path.

Same Day Dentistry: My Different Path

One of the primary reasons I took my own path through Same Day Dentistry was my conscience. I could no longer work in an environment that I felt prized financial gain over the needs—particularly the *immediate* needs —of my patients.

But another major reason was that I felt corporate dentistry was taking a field I was passionate about and reducing it to a cookie-cutter formula rather than a flexible method.

As dentists, we're probably more prone than others to find a regimented formula attractive; that's how we got through dental school, after all. Add A to B and you'll get C. That gets you your passing grades. That gets you your license. That unlocks a whole new set of protocols to follow. There's a reason why those protocols are in place, of course, and I'm not advocating throwing all of that out and practicing in a space free from regulation and order. It's just that I wanted something more, and I found that in Same Day Dentistry. It's not an exact science and I've far from perfected it, but I can tell you that now, several years into walking my different path, I've been able to strike a balance between protocol and philosophy. That's why I call Same Day Dentistry a "method," rather than a "formula." It leaves room for the rules and regulations, of course, and it leaves room for scalability and for business acumen, all the while, letting the true heart of the dentist at the helm shine through.

I've found that many dentists with whom I discuss my Same Day Dentistry practice, want a quick answer—again, usually in the form of a formula.

"Can't you give me something I can take home and implement on Monday morning?" they want to know. I have to disappoint them; the answer is "No." There are some procedures—particularly when it comes to efficiency and billing—that can be scaled up, of course. But largely, the process of creating a Same Day Dentistry office is done through the filter of individuals and the strengths of those individuals. A Same Day Dentistry office is built around an individual dentist (or team of dentists, as the case may be), the assistants, and the staff. It's built around individual strengths and weaknesses, whatever those might be—charisma, charm, experience, extroversion, or even introversion! The idea that this process can't be reduced to a formula or process may be slightly uncomfortable for someone who is used to the formulaic feel of a corporate office. But the dividends it pays are absolutely worth any discomfort that might arise.

One of the reasons why it's so important to me that Same Day Dentistry remain a method rather than a formula goes back to my own experiences that drew me to starting a Same Day Dentistry practice in the first place. I had spent the better part of three decades trying to follow the formulas of supposed gurus, consultants, and master dentists. I'd thought that what was working so well for them would also work for me. But part of being true to myself was recognizing that that wasn't the case. In order to continue to be true to myself, I want to continue to spread the Same Day Dentistry gospel, in a sense, but with the important caveat that you should feel free to take what works for you and leave the rest. (As long as that "rest" doesn't include the heart and soul of Same Day Dentistry: transparency and authenticity, of course!)

Same Day Dentistry Makes Cents: Why the Financials Win Out over Corporate

I could go on for what I imagine would be hundreds of pages about the ethical and emotional benefits of opening a Same Day Dentistry practice, as opposed to continuing to languish inside a corporate environment, but I don't want to give the impression that financials simply aren't important to me, or to any other dentist. Again, unlike the reputation that we seem to have amassed in the public eye, dentists are people who work for a living, who don't necessarily want to sink all of their profits into a faster car, a bigger boat, or a nicer house. Just like our typical patients, we're concerned with making a stable life for ourselves and for our families. For the vast majority of us, and for the employees who depend on our success for their livelihood as well, making ends meet from year to year is not optional; it's a necessity.

The bottom line varies from dentist to dentist and office to office, but among my colleagues who have joined me in implementing a Same Day Dentistry concept into their existing dental practice, the financial rewards are clear. Particularly for dentists who are already making their baseline income to cover their operating costs, the considerable income that results from same-day procedures can feel like the proverbial icing on the cake. I hesitate to give you specific numbers because this isn't a formula and results vary from practice to practice, but I know that in my own practice, I've been able to add *$2,000 to $4,000 of daily productivity* through implementing the Same Day Dentistry concept. I don't know about you, but that kind of control and fiscal solvency feels pretty good to me—particularly after I felt undervalued and underpaid in the corporate dental world for so many years. I know that in my area, there are many plumbers and electricians who make more per hour than dentists in the corporate structure do. This is not to say that plumbers and electricians don't deserve to make a living wage, but rather, that a health-care professional who has invested up to hundreds of thousands of dollars in his skill set and education is going to feel pretty underappreciated by comparison.

Because the Same Day Dentistry model must have buy-in from your whole team to ensure success, it follows that the entire team should also have an incentive for that success to unfold. In my office, that incentive is financial as well as philosophical. My team shares in the profit; so the more business we do, the better they do. But unlike the corporate-dentistry culture, we don't have a culture of salesmanship, of pressure. It's just simply the fruits of our labor of love: fitting more patients into *that same day* to find solutions to their problems on *that same day.*

As wonderful as all of this has been for me and my team, the financial freedom of Same Day Dentistry can be anxiety-producing for dentists who are looking for a simple calculation when it comes to the income side of their ledger. Same Day Dentistry is not as simple, not as neat, as corporate dentistry. I like to think of it as a controlled chaos—one that requires more thinking on your feet, to be sure, but one that is infinitely more interesting and challenging. If you find the idea of giving up control of some of the day-to-day realities— leaving room for those last-minute patient emergencies, for example—stimulating and adrenaline-producing, then Same Day Dentistry might be for you. And with that lack of control comes gaining a completely different type of control: control of your practice, control of your mission, and control of creating an environment in which the patient comes first.

You Can't Beat the Triple Win

It's easy to be an evangelist for a system like Same Day Dentistry when I think about all the good it's done for me and my staff. But what makes it even *more* of a pleasure to sing the praises of Same Day Dentistry is what this method does for my patients. As I said earlier, patients are absolutely the most important part of that terrific Triple Win.

I recall in particular a patient named Don who came to us after starting his dental treatment at a local corporate chain. This patient was what we call "cost-sensitive." He had a strict budget, and he assumed that a corporate chain would be able to perform the same services for less money—kind of like how a big-box store can afford to offer huge discounts to the customer. But if something seems too good to be true, it probably is, and this patient realized that quickly. It turned out that we were able to offer him services at less than the cost of our chain competition, mostly because we pass along to our patients the savings that result from our efficiencies, rather than using that money to line our own coffers. And from a quality-of-care standpoint, I can tell you that this patient felt more heard and more taken care of in our office. It wasn't that we were offering services that the corporate chain wasn't. It wasn't that we were offering radically different technology than that of the corporate chain. Instead, it was that priceless feeling of trust and transparency that our approach engenders.

In the spirit of transparency, I should emphasize once more that the patient wasn't the only one who came out on top in this scenario. I got into this profession to help people, to solve problems, to make people feel heard and, ultimately, feel better.

I didn't become a dentist to worry about how I was supporting salespeople in making their quotas. I certainly didn't become a dentist to pull in a big salary or drive a flashy car. And when I have the privilege of serving a patient like Don, a patient who had pressing problems that needed to be solved, I'm reminded of why I'm really here, and why I've built Same Day Dentistry.

There are times when conventional dentists will argue that upselling a patient like Don who might have an immediate issue but who also has underlying issues that could wait until later is the most productive thing to do. Those dentists might argue that it would make the best return on their investment of time with Don to upsell him into replacing his old silver fillings while they were in there rooting out an infection, for instance. But in my case, that's not what I'm looking to do. I'm looking to get an immediate issue solved first. I'm not looking at return on investment, because I know I've already structured my business to take care of my costs. I'm just looking at Don: Don's mouth, Don's smile, and Don's health.

In many cases, it's very easy to look at a vulnerable patient and forget that his or her pain is paramount. Faced with the pressure to make payroll, dentists might easily slip into sales pitches—and for a vulnerable patient who is in pain, who is lacking in knowledge of what he really needs and what he could do with putting off, it's can be easy for him to slip into agreeing to expensive procedures or intimidating treatment plans. There are absolutely acute situations out there, but after thirty-plus years of practicing dentistry, I can say without hesitation that, for the most part, many of the things that are being sold to these patients as immediate necessities are actually subacute needs that can be dealt with as time and budget allow. In a Same Day Dentistry office, you're able to be honest with yourself —and with your patients—about that reality.

considering your options; I did that for plenty of years. But if you're not serious about making the commitment to change that a shift to Same Day Dentistry requires, then you're better off waiting for another time to make that shift—if you make it at all.

I've put in over three decades of learning the skills and honing the procedural tactics that it takes to make my Same Day Dentistry office run smoothly. That kind of skill won't come overnight, even if you're far more talented than I am! The fact remains: the Same Day Dentistry approach isn't something in which you can just dabble. You have to be all in to gain the critical mass of skills that you'll need to make your Same Day Dentistry office run efficiently and effectively.

Take, for example, the CAD/CAM crown-design technology that we use in my office. It's not enough to invest in the latest-and-greatest technology; you truly have to train with it and learn its ins and outs. And that not only takes a financial commitment, but also, a commitment of significant time and energy. With my nine years of training in techniques including CAD/Cam crown-design technology, I have the ability to deliver a finished crown to a patient *within two hours.* That's the kind of turnaround that enables me to deliver on the Same Day Dentistry promise. What's more, I have the capability and the experience to take a patient in the morning and give him or her a complete smile makeover—six or eight front teeth finished—by the end of the day.

Not everyone has the equipment or the training to do that; that comes with time and tenacity. And that brings us to the final question on your list of things to brainstorm: **"Do I believe in myself?"** You never know what you can accomplish unless you aspire to try. I never would have gotten to this point without a story full of stumbles and missteps; it's important to remember that those same stumbles and missteps are an integral part of the journey to success. Had I not believed in myself that I could truly offer same-day services in my practice, had I not pushed myself to find a way to make that happen, I certainly wouldn't be writing this book.

So if you're serious, and if you believe in yourself, then by all means, read on.

Talking Tech: Investments You Can Expect to Make When Switching to Same Day Dentistry

With the right dentist and the right team, same-day procedures like root canals, extractions, and fillings are fairly standard. But those aren't the real revenue generators. To tap into those kinds of procedures with the sort of skill and efficiency that patients will associate with a truly satisfying Same

Day Dentistry experience, you're going to have to be willing to spend some money to make money. I've enumerated two areas below that can give you a pretty good place to start when it comes to judging what types of technology and techniques you'll need to invest in as a Same Day dentist.

Crowns

At baseline, dentists who want to practice Same Day Dentistry have to be willing to make investments that will allow them to deliver a crown in a day. The cost for the equipment itself will total over $100,000, but this is to say nothing of the time you will need to invest in your own education in order to get as proficient and efficient as possible. And you have to be wiling to be tenacious when it comes to sharpening your skills. It's entirely possible that when you start out, you won't be able to complete a crown in two hours. Perhaps, for you, that procedure will start out taking four hours or so. But even that is a big leap from "someday" dentistry; you're still doing the crown in the same day. As long as you continue to aspire to be more efficient and thus, more profitable, you're headed in the right direction. Increasing efficiencies looks different for everyone, but again, at baseline, it will mean streamlining procedures, whittling down your equipment to the most essential of the very best available, having an organized and systematic approach to the process, and maintaining consistent execution.

In my office, as with many of these procedures, I've found that it's possible to delegate many steps, particularly the preparatory steps such as scanning, to a hygienist or assistant, given that he or she is the *right* hygienist or assistant. Not everyone will be up for the challenge, and that's OK. We all have our strengths that we bring to the table. My point is simply that the more you can delegate, and the more you can bring your supporting team up to speed on what you're doing, the better opportunity you have to complete procedures like crowns at a continuously quicker clip.

Going Digital

Given my emphasis on what's right for the individual dentist, I usually hesitate to make any sweeping pronouncements like this, but I've found this one warrants an exception. I would caution you against pursuing a Same Day Dentistry operation if you aren't willing and able to commit to having a 100 percent computerized office—or at the very least, have a good start in that direction. This means your record-keeping and front-of-office functionality of course, but it goes beyond that, back into the dental suites. Large-screen, high-definition display monitors are absolutely essential for the kind of streamlined discussions and patient preparation that occur with Same Day Dentistry.

Another large investment that's of a piece with the digital displays and seamlessly integrated charting technology is the investment in high-end imaging devices. In my case, this was another $100,000+ investment in the form of a digital panoramic X-ray machine with the three-dimensional cone-beam capacity. This technology allows me to get the best images possible to support my doing the best work I can do, all the while creating a far more comfortable experience for the patient during exams and X-rays than the standard bitewing-film method allows.

Many dentists tend to look at purchasing this kind of X-ray technology as a cost they can offset by charging fees for the exam and the film. In our office, we waive the fees, believing, instead, that it represents an investment in patient care, rather than a cost to us. The cost to recoup is minimal when you factor in all of the satisfied patients—and same-day treatment cash flow— we've been able to accrue in part because of the high-caliber technology we've got helping us out. I stand a much better chance of triaging a patient's needs appropriately if I can clearly see those needs too, meaning that we almost always get a clear view of what problems are "Same Day" problems and what problems can be considered "someday" problems—or, in some cases, which cases need to be referred to a specialist.

Finally, the three-dimensional-imaging capabilities that I have in my office allow me to do another popular procedure more accurately and quickly than I would be able to otherwise. Implants and the creation of artificial roots are simply not possible with anything less than a 3-D image. My X-rays allow me to see precisely the length, width, and placement of the implant, giving me a level of control and accuracy that saves my office *and* the patient the time and money involved in coming back for a procedure that often is stretched over the course of multiple visits. Same-day implants have been a wonderful revenue generator for our office, and I can say without reservation that the patients love the idea that on the same day they have a tooth extracted, they can walk out of the office with an artificial root or implant. I simply could not provide this service safely, comfortably, and confidently without access to a three-dimensional image of the patient's jawbone.

Investing in the Future: Hiring My Junior Associate

Unlike my crown machine and the updated X-ray technology, my most recent investment wasn't a piece of equipment at all. It was my junior associate. In this regard, I look at him more as just an investment for our office, though he certainly is exactly that. Rather, I look at him as an investment in the future of the Same Day Dentistry philosophy—part of leaving that legacy for other dentists to pick up.

I can't help but think that some of my colleagues saw that I was looking for a junior dentist—a long and not inexpensive process—and thought, *Charlie must be ready to retire!* Let me disabuse them—and you!—of that notion right here, right now: far from it. I brought on a junior dentist in part so that I could continue to deliver on my promise of Same Day Dentistry care to my patients as our practice continues to expand. But more than that, I brought on a junior dentist as part of a process to pass the torch on to the next generation of dentists. Many of these individuals, much like my new junior associate, haven't been exposed to a world of dentistry where self-actualization, profitability, and patient care are all possible. As we discussed in the last chapter, many of them are withering away in corporate dental environments, struggling to make ends meet and reap any returns on *their* very large investment: their dental education.

Instead of just being another person propagating the old way of doing dentistry, I am striving to leave a different mark. In training this junior dentist (and hopefully, others to come) in the ways of Same Day Dentistry, I'm optimistic that I can nurture individuals who have compassion, patience, humility, and—most of all—the desire to serve their communities. Ultimately, I hope to teach this younger generation the virtues of being transparent and truthful. I hope to spare them decades of questioning and soul-searching, of wondering if they'd wandered down the wrong path.

It's important to emphasize that this individual is an *investment*. Looking at a junior dentist as an investment as opposed to just another warm body to take on some of the workload is the first step in crafting not only a successful collegial relationship, but in utilizing your entire team to its potential. Typically, I found that in past offices I practiced in, a junior dentist was just another plug-and-play device— someone to take on more procedures and increase the cash flow. In my office, I'm pleased to say, we're looking at the bigger picture: utilizing that person's drive, attitude, personality, and, of course, dental skills, to enhance the practice overall.

In this effort, I must admit that I enjoy the selfish pleasure of seeing my work continue for generations. And hopefully, my junior dentist and anyone else who comes to study by my side has the pleasure of seeing his or her career blossom in a way he or she would have had a hard time imagining before. But it all comes back to the top of that Triple Win: the patients.

Because I believe that by continuing to practice the same rote, corporate, and profit-driven dentistry that our patients have come to expect, we're doing a disservice to the profession and doing a disservice to patients. I've met so many patients who have felt so skeptical, so abused, so gun-shy about even entering a dental office for a routine cleaning because of how they've been treated in the past. I know that I don't have all the answers, and I hope to continue learning as well, but I do know that I want to help provide a larger solution for this kind of negative experience. My plans are not too grand: I'm hoping that, by the time I'm no longer in circulation, there will be at least a dozen dentists who can take my place in my community, providing the Same Day Dentistry Triple Win over and over again. And if those dentists can continue to reach out to one another, continue to educate one another, I will have absolutely served my community in a better way than if had I just stuck with the status quo.

CHAPTER TEN

Join the Same Day Dentistry Revolution!

I f you were a patient of mine, I know just how this next part would go. I would ask you how you're feeling. I would ask if there are any adjustments that we need to make to get you feeling as close to 100 percent as possible. I would ask if you had any questions, if there was anything further I could do to help.

But this—talking *to* you, rather than *with* you, from within these pages—this is new for me. In the spirit of being true to myself, then, I think I'll stick with what I know.

I have a pretty good idea of how you might be feeling, and of some of the motivations you might have had in turning to this book. You might be looking to expand your knowledge about the way that dental practices can be structured nowadays. You might just like reading about dentistry! But more than likely, you've picked up this book because you're at a point in your life where you want something more from your profession and your practice. And more than anything, I hope you've been able to find encouragement within these pages.

The Same Day Dentistry revolution is all about finding the courage to raise the bar—not only for yourself, but for your practice and your patients as well. If you've been on the fence at all about making a change, or if you've just been stuck getting along to go along for too many years, I want you to know that there are other possibilities, that the grass can, in fact, be greener on the other side.

It can be tempting to throw yourself whole hog into major changes, especially if you've been frustrated and stagnant for quite some time. On the flip side, it can also be intimidating to take even the smallest step. I've been there; I know. It's never easy to take stock of what you're doing and throw a curveball into the mix, but that's where encouraging voices come in. I'm honored that you've chosen mine to be one of those voices, and I hope that you continue to surround yourself with people who can join in a veritable chorus of can-do spirit!

Whether you're waiting to summon the courage to make the switch to Same Day Dentistry or you're ready to get started in the process, I want you to do me— and yourself—a big favor. If you're starting out, don't put too much pressure on yourself to do it all at once. And if you're still in the contemplative stage, don't become fixated on the idea that you're incapable of small changes. Instead, think about those first steps you can take. Even if you can't devote your entire practice to the Same Day Dentistry concept just yet, weaving in the philosophy I've laid out in this book can be an excellent starting point—not to mention a way to gain greater financial solvency. Ask yourself: Can I devote one room of my practice to Same Day Dentistry patients? Can I devote time to training one dental assistant to help get some of those Same Day Dentistry patients taken care of? Great! You're well on your way.

Part of the benefit of getting your feet wet is that as you make greater financial gains from the Same Day Dentistry segment of your practice, you will be more readily able to make the investments (in technology, time, and staff) that will allow you to expand your services to same-day crowns, implants, etc.

Assuming you have a supportive and versatile staff, you'll also be able to spend time onboarding them into the philosophy and processes of Same Day Dentistry. Remember: your teammates are crucial to your success in a Same Day Dentistry practice, and it's important to invest time and energy in their education.

Still, there are some things you can't train. It might take you a while to get it right, both within yourself and within your team. You can't train things like humility, integrity, or the heart for serving others. But you can certainly hone these qualities in yourself and your staff. You can find those seedlings of truth about how you want to make your mark on the world and you can nurture them and take them to flower.

Flowering is a particularly apt metaphor in this case, because just as our technical skills take us on different paths to different proficiencies, our personalities and our strengths are unique and organic. You don't have to be a mirror image of me to be a success at Same Day Dentistry, just as your team doesn't have to be a mirror image of you. Instead, think about how you can draw out the confidence and inner strengths of yourself and your team members and put those to work. How can you provide a supportive environment for truth and transparency? How can you encourage yourself and your team to be good listeners, to really want to engage with the patients and their pain instead of just ticking them as procedures on a to-do list?

The answers to these questions take time. But finding those answers is far more rewarding than anything I ever did in a traditional practice.

And a word about time. When I say "time" as it pertains to my own journey, it took me about thirty years to get here. It might not take you as long. You might have resources that I didn't, or talents that I didn't, or expertise that I didn't. And this is truly a thrilling proposition for me: that the future generation of dentists won't have to flounder for as long as I did, searching to find my true north. If you're one of those lucky few who is just starting out and already knows where he or she is going, if you're already on your way to becoming a better person, a better servant to your community, and a better practitioner of dentistry, be it through Same Day Dentistry or any other method, my hat is truly off to you.

And to those of you who are like I was—stuck in limbo and unsure of where to go, there's nowhere to go but forward, my friends. And I'm here to tell you that you can get there; *forward* is well within your reach.

I wish I'd had more supportive ears when I was making the jump to Same Day Dentistry, starting my own practice from scratch in Wasilla, Alaska, at the age of fifty-nine. My peers weren't too hopeful about my prospects: "Aren't you getting a little old? Isn't it time to retire?" "Are you crazy!? What if it tanks? What will you do then?" I have to admit, I thought along those same lines myself at points, especially when we opened on that first day without a single patient on the schedule. It may seem like madness to you, but I assure you, there *is* a method here. It might take some soul searching to find your place in it, but you'll get there. That's another fantastic thing about the Same Day Dentistry revolution: there's truly a role for everyone.

Most of our patients probably don't realize this, but as dentists, we don't have the best job in the world. Not only are we struggling to keep up with the changing financial landscape of insurance and the uncertain economic future of any businessperson, but we also have our own crosses to bear when it comes to our profession. We're typically seeing people who don't really want to be in our office. We're faced with the constant rejection that comes with being associated with something that's painful, intimate, and invasive. "No offense, Doc, but I really hate coming to the dentist." "I would rather [insert horrible task here] than go to the dentist." "I'm scared of the dentist." "When I go to the dentist, it feels like I'm paying someone to cause me pain!" Is it any wonder that sometimes it's a struggle to get ourselves excited about getting up and going to work in the morning?

I have to tell you that, more than any other resource, my Same Day Dentistry practice has helped me completely shift my perspective in that regard. I used to be unable to take a compliment, convinced that in order for someone to say something nice about me, there had to be an ulterior motive at hand. But now, after several years of amazing patient reviews that our practice has garnered, I'm a little more used to feeling praiseworthy. I want you to feel that, too—because you are, because you can be, and because you deserve to.

For more information or to get in touch with Dr. Charlie Cole, visit Samedaydentistryrevolution.com

THE SAME DAY DENTISTRY REVOLUTION AT A GLANCE:

A Reference Guide for Readers

Chapter One: Dentistry on the Same Day? What's That All About?

- The Same Day Dentistry revolution is about performing dental procedures on the same day.
- Not all problems can be addressed on the same day, but those that can, should be.

- It's not about making a lengthy treatment plan. It *is* about quality dentistry.
- Transparency is key. We list our procedures, we list the prices, and we don't play games.
- The whole dental team needs to be on board with the Same Day Dentistry mission.
- Our mission is to help patients find solutions that same day, not someday.

Chapter Two: From Someday to Same Day—How the Whole Thing Came About

- I put in over three decades in the dental industry, purchasing and selling conventional practices.
- I also worked as a dentist in a group practice.
- Neither environment was really for me. When I was let go from a practice around Christmastime in 2013, I knew it was time for something completely different.
- I rented a space in an unconventional location—a strip mall in Wasilla, Alaska—and jumped in with both feet.
- It was scary, but three years in, I had a full staff, a full patient roster, and the financial solvency to take my crew on a prepaid all-inclusive trip to Turks and Caicos.

Chapter Three: Why the Traditional Model of Selling Dentistry Is Broken

- The traditional model of dentistry relies on lengthy and expensive treatment plans.
- Same Day Dentistry offices can provide those too, but we always make sure to address the patients' immediate needs, working with them and within their budget.
- Patients don't trust traditional models—partly because they can't afford to, partly because they don't have time to, and partly because they don't feel that those traditional practices are leaving time for their concerns to truly be heard.
- Same Day Dentistry flips the script on that—partly because we don't charge exam fees for the first visit, partly because we address things in an efficient manner, and partly because we really know how to listen!

Chapter Four: The Same Day Dentistry Triple Win: Why Patients, Team, and Doctor All Do Better with Same Day Dentistry

- Patients fare better with Same Day Dentistry because they get quality care in less time for less cost.

- The team does better with Same Day Dentistry because they can share in the profits and be a part of a challenging, fast-paced environment where they are set up to succeed.
- The doctor does better because there's increased financial sustainability, increased productivity, a better relationship with patients, and less opportunity for canceled or missed appointments.

Chapter Five: What to Expect If You're a Same Day Dentistry Patient

- You can expect transparent reviews and information on the web and through word of mouth.
- You can expect an easy-to-get-to location.
- You can expect to be greeted in a waiting-room space that feels more like a living room.
- You can expect one-on-one time with the dentist *before* even getting into the exam chair.
- You can expect top-of-the-line imaging.
- You can expect an easy, transparent discussion with the dentist.
- You can expect a clear treatment plan with no surprise costs.

- You can expect to pay the same if you are paying in cash or with insurance. You should *not* expect credit; it artificially inflates cost and takes advantage of patients.
- You can expect a comfortable visit from start to finish.

Chapter Six: Location, Location, Location . . . Can You Really Practice Dentistry in a Strip Mall?

- Short answer: YES!
- The clothes don't make the man. You don't need a fancy address to practice quality dentistry.
- Your location can serve as your biggest marketing tool.
- An unconventional location might cost less money.
- A street-facing location is more integrated in the community and easier to find, unlike the labyrinth of faceless, generic medical offices.

Chapter Seven: Passing the Savings Along to the Patient— The Economics of Same Day Dentistry

- Same Day dental care should always be affordable.
- We can ensure this because our efficiencies save the office money.

- We can ensure this because our efficiencies save the patient money too.
- By having a consistent handle on our costs, we can calculate appropriate profit margins and pass savings along to the patients.
- Because we have fewer cancellations or missed appointments due to our business model, we can pass those savings along to patients as well.
- Because we don't extend credit, we don't have to deal with agency fees or collection costs, and we can also pass those savings along to the patients.

Chapter Eight: Why Same Day Dentistry Beats Corporate Dentistry Any Day

- Corporate dentistry leaves little room for the individual dentist.
- Corporate dentistry doesn't pay well enough to offset the considerable cost of your education.
- Corporate dentistry doesn't value you as a dentist; they value you as a cog in a sales machine.
- Corporate dentistry encourages upselling and other questionable sales tactics for the benefit of the practice, *not* the patient.

- Same Day Dentistry is the antithesis of corporate dentistry.

Chapter Nine: The Future of Same Day Dentistry

- If you're serious about taking your practice to the Same Day Dentistry level, feel free to visit www.samedaydental.net and get in touch!
- Leaving a legacy is just as important as the here and now. By promoting the Same Day Dentistry philosophy and teaching it to other dentists, we can ensure a world in which quick, quality patient care is accessible to many.

Chapter Ten: Join the Same Day Dentistry Revolution!

- You can do it.
- I know you can.
- So get out there and get going!

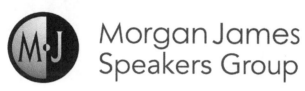
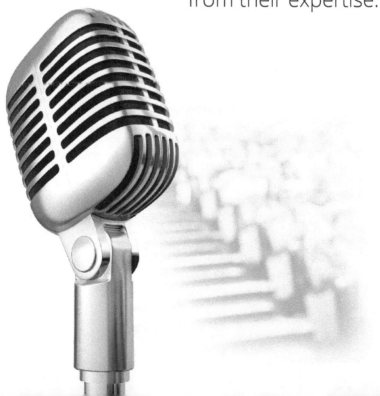

Printed in the USA
CPSIA information can be obtained
at www.ICGtesting.com
JSHW082351140824
68134JS00020B/2017

9 781683 503521